THE SHOPPER'S GUIDE TO

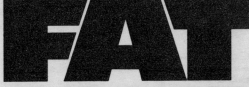

IN YOUR FOOD

A CARRY-ALONG GUIDE TO THE FAT, CALORIES, AND FAT PERCENTAGES IN BRAND NAME FOODS

KAREN J. BELLERSON

Avery Publishing Group
Garden City Park, New York

SOURCES

Food manufacturers and processors direct, as well as their product labels.

United States Department of Agriculture Handbook No. 8, revised, "Composition of Foods, Raw, Processed, Prepared," sections 8-1 through 8-22; Agriculture Handbook No. 456, "Nutritive Value of American Foods In Common Units"; Home and Garden Bulletin No. 232, "Nutrition and Your Health: Dietary Guidelines for Americans."

Individual fast food chains.

Cover designers: Rudy Shur, Evan Schwartz, and Bill Gonzalez
In-house editors: Bonnie Freid, Joanne Abrams, Elaine Will Sparber, and Marie Caratozzolo
Typesetters: Kerri Matheson and Bonnie Freid

ISBN 0-89529-610-1

Printed in the United States of America

10 9 8 7 6 5 4

Introduction

Countless studies continue to prove that there is a very real relationship between our diet and the risk of developing a life-threatening disease. In response to these findings, the United States Department of Agriculture has replaced the Four Basic Food Groups of milk, meat, vegetables and fruits, and breads and cereals with the new Food Guide Pyramid (see Figure 1).

Notice that fats, oils, and sweets are the smallest part of the new Food Guide Pyramid. This new pyramid reflects advice from all the major health organizations recommending a diet consisting of 55 to 60 percent carbohydrates, 15 percent protein, and *no more than 30 percent fat.* There are some who feel that only 25 percent or less of our calories should come from fat, in order to lower our risk of heart disease and some kinds of cancer.

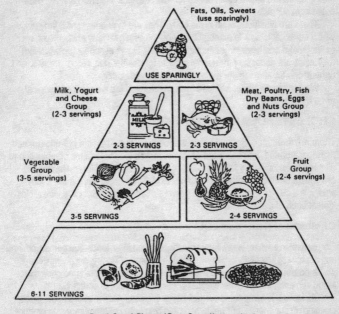

Figure 1. The Food Guide Pyramid.

FAT IS REQUIRED BY THE BODY

The fact is that we need some fat in our diets. Adults need a minimum daily intake of 15 to 25 grams of dietary fat to meet the body's needs. (Children under the age of two years should not have their dietary fat restricted, however, because of the possible interference with their development.)

Our bodies use fat in numerous ways—ways in which most of us are unaware. We use fat in manufacturing antibodies to fight disease. Fats act as carriers for the fat-soluble vitamins A, D, E, and K. Fat deposits cushion, protect, and hold in place vital organs such as the kidneys, heart, and liver. Fat is the body's insulation against environmental temperature changes and is what gives the body its shape. While fat is one of the three nutrient energy sources, it also aids in digestion by slowing down the stomach's secretions of hydrochloric acid, which is what produces that satisfying feeling of fullness after a meal. So, as you can see, fat should not be totally eliminated from our diets!

There are two types of fat in the body. They are the nonessential fatty acids, which our body is able to manufacture, and the essential fatty acids, which we cannot make and have to get through our diets. These essential (unsaturated) fatty acids are necessary for normal growth; for healthy skin, blood, arteries, and nerves; and for keeping our metabolism running smoothly.

We can get all the fat we need from unsaturated fat; there is no biological need for saturated fat!

CHOLESTEROL AND DIETARY FAT

There are three main types of fats in the foods we eat. They are polyunsaturated, monounsaturated, and saturated. Most processed foods contain a combination of all three kinds of dietary fat. The percentage of each type of fat is what makes one food a healthier choice than another food. While cholesterol is not a fatty acid, it is a fat-like substance and is often referred to as a "fat." Let's take a closer look at each of these substances.

Cholesterol (HDL and LDL)

Cholesterol is a white, waxy, fatty substance found in all foods that come from animal sources, particularly organ meats such as brains, kidney, and liver. Because plants do not have the ability to manufacture cholesterol, there is no cholesterol found in plants; this includes oils that come from vegetable sources.

Cholesterol is essential to our well-being. We don't need a lot of it in our blood, clogging up our arteries, but we do need it to help build cell membranes, to produce hormones (estrogen, progesterone, and testosterone), and to manufacture bile acids that are needed to eliminate excess cholesterol from the body. About 75 percent of the cholesterol found in our body (all our body needs) is manufactured in our liver, even if we don't eat animal products; the other 25 percent comes from our diet.

The cholesterol manufactured by our liver is carried through our bloodstream by LDLs (low-density lipoproteins). High levels of LDLs in the bloodstream can result in clogged arteries, causing high blood pressure, stroke, or heart disease. This is why LDL is referred to as the "bad" cholesterol or, as I refer to it, the "lethal" cholesterol. LDL levels can be reduced through proper diet.

Now we come to the HDLs (high-density lipoproteins), the "good" cholesterol (I refer to it as the "healthy" cholesterol). HDLs carry excess cholesterol from different body tissues to the liver, where it is metabolized by the liver and then processed through the intestines and eliminated from the body. High levels of these HDLs are correlated with a decreased risk of coronary heart disease. HDL levels can be raised through regular exercise.

Polyunsaturated Fats

Polyunsaturated fats are found in most foods, including certain fish (Omega-3), but mainly in nuts, oils from plants, seeds, and soybeans (Omega-6). These fats are liquid at room temperature. Polyunsaturated fats reduce blood cholesterol, but an excess may lower the protective "good" cholesterol, HDL. (Some studies speculate that there is a link between polyunsaturates and breast cancer.)

Foods with higher contents of polyunsaturated fats include the following:

Bagels	Fish	Salad Dressings
Barbecue Sauce	Lentils	Seeds
Bread (French, Italian, Raisin, Oatmeal, Pumpernickel, and Rye)	Nuts (Pine, Walnuts, and Brazil)	Soybeans
	Popcorn (air popped)	Squash
		Sweet Potatoes
Chickpeas (Garbanzo Beans)	Potato Chips	Tuna Salad
	Potato Salad	Tofu
Corn Chips	Refried Beans	Vegetable and Nut Oils

Monounsaturated Fats

Monounsaturated fats are found in most foods, but mainly in vegetable and nut oils such as olive, peanut, and canola (rapeseed). These fats are also liquid at room temperature. Monounsaturated fats reduce total blood cholesterol while not having the side effect of lowering the protective "good" cholesterol, HDL.

Be aware that both polyunsaturated and monounsaturated fats can be hydrogenated. Hydrogenation is a process of adding hydrogen to an oil in order to make it more solid at room temperature so that it can be used in processing foods such as baked goods, non-dairy creamers, and whipped toppings. Hydrogenation of unsaturated fats makes them saturated. When reading product labels, watch for the words "hydrogenated" or "partially hydrogenated."

The following foods have higher contents of monounsaturated fats. Those foods marked with an asterisk (*) are also higher in saturated fats.

Almonds
Animal Fats
Avocados
Beef* (leaner cuts)
Biscuits
Bread* (most types—read your labels)
Brownies
Cake* (most types)
Chicken
Cookies
Croissants
Donuts
Eggs*

Fruitcake
Gingerbread
Lard*
Margarine (stick)
Muffins*
Nuts (Hazelnuts, Cashews, Chestnuts, Macadamia, Peanuts, Pecans, and Pistachio)
Oatmeal
Ocean Perch
Pastry* (includes pie crust)
Peanut Butter

Pies* (most types)
Popcorn (popped in vegetable oil)
Pork
Sausage* (most types)
Shortening (vegetable)
Spaghetti (with tomato sauce)
Taco
Veal* (leaner cuts)
Vegetable and Nut Oils

Saturated Fats

Foods containing saturated fats include all meat and dairy products. The tropical oils, coconut, palm, and palm kernel, although from plant origin, are also high in saturated fat. Cocoa butter, the oil used in making chocolate, is also a highly saturated fat source. Use powdered cocoa instead in all your recipes calling for choco late. Saturated fats are generally solid at room temperature. Remember that saturated fats—more than dietary cholesterol—raise total blood cholesterol.

The following foods have higher contents of saturated fats. For other foods higher in these fats, see the list of high-monounsaturated-fat foods, as those foods marked with asterisks (*) are also high in saturated fats.

Beef (fattier cuts)
Butter
Cake (snack, most types, and those with chocolate frosting)

Cheese (most types)
Cheesecake
Chili (with beef)
Chocolate
Cocoa butter

Cocoa mixes
Coconut (and all coconut products)
Cottage cheese (4 percent fat)
Cream

Custard (baked)
Eggnog
Fried Foods (using
 saturated oils)
Granola
Gravy (brown—
 packaged)
Hot Dogs
Ice Cream
Ice Milk
Lamb
Luncheon Meats Malts
Milk (whole, 2, & 1%)

Non-Dairy
 Creamers
Non-Dairy Whipped
 Cream
Pies (Cream)
Pizza
Popcorn
Pork (fattier cuts)
Puddings
Pumpkin
Sauces (Bear-
 naise, Hollandaise
Seaweed

Shakes
Soups (most
 cream types)
Sour Cream
Turkey (dark meat)
Turkey (self-
 basting)
Veal (fattier cuts)
Vegetable and
 Nut Oils
Yogurt (made from
 whole milk solids)

GUIDELINES FOR REDUCING THE FAT IN YOUR DIET

As I mentioned earlier, fat is needed for healthy body functions and should not be totally eliminated from our diets. The Surgeon General's Report on Nutrition and Health (1988) conveyed, "Adults need a minimum daily intake of 15 to 25 grams of fat to meet these necessities."

The American Heart Association; the American-Health Foundation; the American Cancer Society; the National Heart, Lung, and Blood Institute; the National Center for Nutrition and Dietetics; the American Diabetes Association; and the Surgeon General all recommend that no more than 30 percent of our daily calories should come from fat, and no more than one-third of those fats (or 10 percent of our daily calories) should be saturated fats! Below, I will show you how to calculate this 30 percent and even 20 percent (in case you want to lower your fat intake even more).

FAT CALORIES *ARE* DIFFERENT!

Fat calories are indeed different from carbohydrate and protein calories. That difference is very important for us to understand, because we can actually replace fat with more carbohydrates and protein and still be eating fewer calories! Yes, it's true!

Why? Not only does fat have 9 calories per gram, while carbohydrates and protein have only 4 calories each per gram, but the way our body metabolizes dietary fat is different from the way it processes carbohydrates or protein. Dietary fat is very similar in chemical composition to our body fat, so it takes less energy to convert it to body fat. It takes only 3 percent of the calories in the fat we eat to turn that food into body fat, while it takes at least 25 percent of the carbohydrate and protein calories we eat to convert them into body fat. What does this mean? It means that reducing the fat in our diets is not only the most healthy way to eat, it is also an excellent way to control our weight! Maybe there really is something to that old saying about fat, "You eat it, you wear it! Remember, though, that if you eat more calories than your body needs, regardless of the nutrient providing these calories, the excess will be stored as body fat.

FAT GRAM BUDGET FORMULA

Fortunately, if you have decided to reduce your dietary fat, there is a simple formula that will let you know exactly how many fat grams you should allow yourself on a daily basis. To find out your maximum daily allowance, multiply your daily calorie intake by .30, and divide that total by 9 (there are 9 calories in each gram of fat). For a daily intake of 1,500 calories, your equation would look like this:

$$1500 \times .30 + 9 = 50 \text{ OR } 1500 \times .30 = 450.00 + 9 = 50$$

Of course, to calculate your daily fat gram budget, you need to know your daily calorie intake. To find this out, if you don't already know, just use *The Shopper's Guide to the Fat in Your Food* to keep a diary for three or four days. This will help you determine more precisely your actual daily calorie intake. Write down everything you eat or drink for these days, add up the totals, then divide by the number of days you kept track. Remember that just because you have budgeted X amount of fat grams for the day, you don't need to eat that amount of fat. Just make sure not to go over the budget!

So you will have a means of comparison, I have taken the guesswork out of it for you by listing the fat gram budgets for the following daily calorie intakes. The following table shows both 30-percent and 20-percent maximum daily fat gram budgets.

Daily Calorie Intake	Fat Grams Allowed 20%	30%	Daily Calorie Intake	Fat Grams Allowed 20%	30%
1,200	27	40	2,200	49	73
1,300	29	43	2,300	51	76
1,400	31	46	2,400	53	80
1,500	33	50	2,500	56	83
1,600	36	53	2,600	58	86
1,700	38	56	2,700	60	90
1,800	40	60	2,800	62	93
1,900	42	63	2,900	64	96
2,000	44	66	3,000	67	100
2,100	47	70			

Note that this data has been rounded off by dropping all decimal places. This chart begins at 1,200 calories, as it is not recommended for anyone to eat fewer than 1,200 calories (for women) or 1,500 calories (for men) in order to meet her or his daily nutritional needs.

HOW TO USE THIS BOOK

The Shopper's Guide to the Fat in Your Food is meant to be used as a take along guide while you are shopping at your local market. As you shop for and prepare low-fat foods, this book will be an invaluable source of information. For a more in-depth and comprehensive reference book, *The Complete & Up-to-Date Fat Book* contains over 25,000 listings of foods found in markets and fast foods establishments, in the same easy-to-follow format.

Serving amount, fat grams, total calories, and percentage of fat calories are provided for every product listed. In most cases, the foods are listed alphabetically for ready-reference. Some foods, where appropriate, are listed in groups, i.e., Frozen Entree/Dinner, Mexican Food, Oriental Food, etc.

Since cereals and soups are frequently prepared with milk, quick-reference charts for adding milk can be found in these sections. Also, because when we use oil in our food preparation it's important that we choose the least saturated oil available to us, I have prepared a chart on page 51, showing the breakdown by percentage of saturated, polyunsaturated, and monounsaturated fat contents of the most commonly used fats and oils.

As far as style, the book is organized with main headings for food capitalized and bold, and subheadings smaller (also capitalized and bold) with solid boxes before them. Descriptions of foods are upper/lower case, with brand names in parentheses. If you are unable to find a particular food, look for the listing of a similar food. The nutritional data should be close, if not exact, for any product not listed. When doing this, make sure you are comparing the same serving size. Also, be sure you are comparing weight measure against weight measure and volume measure against volume measure. Note that all cooked vegetable amounts are drained of liquid, unless otherwise noted.

You will find *The Shopper's Guide to the Fat in Your Food* a valuable companion as you begin to take control of your eating habits. And you will discover that adopting a low-fat lifestyle reaps many rewards—rewards such as more energy, better sleep, lower grocery bills, more control over your weight, and, perhaps most important, radiant health!

Food and Description	Amount	Fat Grams	Total Calories	% Fat Calories
ALMOND				
(Eagle)honey roasted	1 oz	12	150	72%
(Planters)/blanched sliced	1 oz	15	170	79%
APPLE				
(Del Monte) sliced	2 oz	0	140	0
(Nature's Favorite) Apple Chips	1 oz	5	120	38%
(Sun Maid) chunks	2 oz	0	150	0
APPLE CIDER				
Bottled/(Indian Summer)	6 oz	0	100	0
(Tree Top)	6 oz	0	90	0
APPLE JUICE				
Bottled/boxed, or canned				
(Campbell's) Juice Bow l-Apple	6 oz	0	110	0
(Mott's)	8.45 oz	0	124	0
Frozen/(Minute Maid)	6 oz	0	90	0
(Sunkist)	8 oz	0	79	0
APPLESAUCE				
(Del Monte)/Lite	1/2 cup	0	50	0
sweetened	1/2 cup	0	90	0
(Mott's)/cinnamon	4 oz	0	72	0
natural	4 oz	0	44	0
APPLE DUMPLINGS				
(Pepperidge Farm) frozen	3 oz	13	260	45%
ARTICHOKE HEARTS				
canned-marinated/(S & W)	3.5 oz	25	225	100%
ASPARAGUS				
canned/All Green Fancy (S & W)	1/2 cup	0	18	0
fresh-cooked/cuts & tips	1/2 cup	0	22	0
frozen spears (Birds Eye)	3.3 oz	0	25	0
AVOCADO				
California/raw	1	30.79	324	86%
Florida	1	27	340	72%

B

Food and Description	Amount	Fat Grams	Total Calories	% Fat Calories
BACON				
Breakfast Strips/cooked	3 slices	12.5	156	72%
(Eckrich) Sizzlean/cooked	2 slices	8	90	80%
(Oscar Meyer) 93% fat-free	1 oz	1	35	26%
BACON BITS				
(Hormel)	1 Tbs	2	30	60%
(Oscar Meyer)	¼ oz	1	21	43%
BANANA, fresh	1 med.	< 1	101	5%
BEAN, BAKED & VARIETY				
(B&M)/BBQ	~ 1 cup	6	310	17%
Red Kidney	~ 1 cup	7	290	22%
Tomato	~ 1 cup	3	230	12%
Vegetarian	~ 1 cup	2	280	6%
(Green Giant)/baked w/bacon				
& brown sugar	½ cup	1	130	7%
(S&W) Brick Oven	½ cup	2	160	11%
Maple Sugar (S&W)	½ cup	1	150	6%
Pork & Beans/(Campbell's)	8 oz	3	190	14%
(Hunt's)	4 oz	1	140	6%
Vegetarian/(Heinz)	8 oz	1	230	4%
(Libby)	½ cup	1	130	7%

BEEF

(Note: Serving sizes are for cooked beef, unless otherwise stated. "Lean only" means beef trimmed of all separable fat before cooking. "Lean & fat" means untrimmed and cooked or eaten as purchased. Prime cuts have the most fat, Choice cuts less, and Select/Good cuts the least amount of all cuts.)

■ **BEEF CUTS**

Brisket				
Whole/lean & fat-braised	3 oz	27.6	332	75%
Whole/lean only-braised	3 oz	10.9	205	48%
Chuck-pot roast/lean & fat	3 oz	22.5	301	67%
Rib roast or steaks/lean & fat	3 oz	31	364	77%

Food and Description	Amount	Fat Grams	Total Calories	% Fat Calories
Stew meat-boneless/Lean & fat				
Braised or stewed	3 oz	20	279	65%
Lean only/Braised or stewed	3 oz	8	183	39%
Corned Beef/Boneless/Roasted	3 oz	25.8	316	74%
Flank-Lean and fat/Choice				
Braised	3 oz	13	218	54%
Broiled	3 oz	13.9	216	58%
Lean only/Choice-braised	3 oz	11.8	208	51%
Choice-broiled	3 oz	12.7	207	55%
Ground (Note: 4 oz raw ground meat is equal to 3 oz cooked ground meat.)				
Extra lean 15% fat				
Broiled medium	3 oz	13.9	215	58%
Broiled well-done	3 oz	13	225	52%
Extra Lean 10% Fat/Raw	4 oz	11	202	49%
Broiled well-done	3 oz	9.6	186	46%
(Healthy Choice) Regular/Raw	4 oz	30	351	77%
Broiled medium	3 oz	17.6	246	64%
Broiled well-done	3 oz	16.5	248	60%
London Broil, 100% lean	3 oz	6	167	32%
Rib/Whole/lean & fat				
Choice-broiled	3 oz	26	313	75%
Good-roasted	3 oz	24.9	306	73%
Lean only Choice-broiled	3 oz	11.5	198	52%
Sirloin Ground (Chef's Grind)				
10% Fat	3 oz	8	140	51%
Steak/Porterhouse/lean & fat				
Choice-broiled	3 oz	18	254	64%
T-bone/lean & fat Choice-broiled	3 oz	20.9	276	68%
Lean only Choice-broiled	3 oz	8.8	182	44%
Tenderloin/Choice-broiled	3 oz	15	230	59%
Choice-roasted	3 oz	19	262	65%
BEEF DISHES				
Beef Pot Pie Frozen/(Banquet)	7 oz	33	510	58%
(Swanson)	7 oz	20	380	47%
Beef Stew/Canned				
(Bounty) vegetable	7.6 oz	3	144	19%
(Healthy Choice)	7.5 oz	2	140	13%

Food and Description	Amount	Fat Grams	Total Calories	% Fat Calories
(Libby's) vegetable	7.5 oz	5	160	28%
Frozen/(Banquet)	7 oz	5	140	32%
Microwaveable/(Lunch Bucket)	8.5 oz	6	170	32%
Beefaroni (Chef Boyardee)	7 oz	6	200	27%
BISCUITS				
Frozen (Bridgeford)	1	6	190	28%
Mix/Baking mix (Krusteaz) 2" dia	1	4	110	33%
Refrigerated				
Big Country Butter (Pillsbury)	1	4	100	36%
Butter (Pillsbury)	1	< 1	50	9%
Southern Style (Hungry Jack)	1	4	80	45%
BRAN				
Oat/(Golden Harvest)	1 oz	2	90	20%
(Quaker)	½ cup	3.8	165	21%
Rice/(Golden Harvest)	½ cup	8	120	60%
Rite Bran/(Uncle Ben's)	½ cup	9	100	81%
Toasted Wheat (Kretchmer)	⅓ cup	2	60	30%
BREAD				
Box mix-Quick (Pillsbury)				
Banana	1/12 loaf	6	170	32%
Date	1/12 loaf	3	160	17%
Bran	1 slice	2.9	110	24%
Bran'nola/Country Oat	1 slice	3	90	30%
Date Nut/Deli Rye	1 slice	1	70	13%
Raisin Cinnamon Swirl	1 slice	2	80	23%
Egg	1 slice	2.6	75	31%
Granola (Country Hearth)	1 slice	1	70	13%
Multi-Bran (Roman Meal)	1 slice	1	64	14%
Oat (Roman Meal)	1 slice	1	70	13%
Oat & Honey/(Pepperidge Farm)	1 slice	2	65	28%
Pita-6 ½" dia	1 slice	.5	165	3%
Pumpernickel (Pepperidge Farm)	1 slice	1	80	11%
Pumpernickel-Rye/(Earth Grains)	1 slice	1	70	13%
Raisin (Pepperidge Farm)	2 slices	4	180	20%
Rye/(Pepperidge Farm) Family	1 slice	1	80	11%
(Weight Watchers)				
Cinnamon Raisin	1 slice	1	60	15%
Rye	1 slice	< 1	40	11%

Food and Description	Amount	Fat Grams	Total Calories	% Fat Calories
thin slice	2 slices	< 1	40	6%
White	1 slice	1	65	14%
Sandwich (Pepperidge Farm)	2 slices	2	130	14%
Toasting (Pepperidge Farm)	1 slice	1	90	10%
Whole Grain (Roman Meal)	1 slice	1	66	14%
Whole Wheat	1 slice	1	65	14%
(Wonder)				
Rye Breads				
Beefsteak Hearty Rye, Mild Rye, Onion Rye, Soft Rye, Wheatberry Rye	1 slice	1	70	13%
Wonder Rye	1 slice	1	70	13%
Wheat Breads				
Beefsteak Hearty Wheat	1 slice	1	70	13%
(Home Pride)	1 slice	1	70	13%
White Breads				
Home Pride Butter Top	1 slice	1	70	13%
Wonder Thin Sliced	1 slice	1	50	18%
BREAD CRUMBS				
(Contadina)-seasoned	1 cup	3.6	426	6%
(Progresso)/plain & italian	2 Tbs	< 1	60	8%
BREAD STICKS				
(Pillsbury) Refrigerated soft	1	2	100	18%
(Stella D'Oro)/Onion	1	1	40	23%
Pizza	1	1	43	21%
Plain	1	1	41	22%
BREAD STUFFIN				
dry	1 cup	31	500	56%
moist	1 cup	26	420	56%
BREAKFAST BAR				
(Carnation) Breakfast Bars				
Chocolate chip	1 bar	11	200	50%
Peanut butter crunch	1 bar	10	190	47%
(Health Valley)/Fat-Free Fruit	1 bar	< 1	95	5%
Fruit & Fitness Energy	2 bars	5	200	23%
Oat Bran Fruit/Apples/dates	1 bar	4	150	24%
(Kelloggs) Nutri-grain/'Apple	1 bar	5	150	30%
(Pillsbury) Figurines/Chocolate	1 bar	5	100	45%

Food and Description	Amount	Fat Grams	Total Calories	% Fat Calories
Chocolate peanut butter	1 bar	6	100	54%

BREAKFAST DRINK (NOTE:Drinks and mixes prepared according to package directions.)

Food and Description	Amount	Fat Grams	Total Calories	% Fat Calories
(Alba) Chocolate, Marshmallow, Milk Chocolate, Rich chocolate	1	1	110	8%
(Alba) 77 Fit n Frosty/Choco.	1	1	70	13%
(Carnation) Instant Breakfast Diet-no sugar/Chocolate	1	1	70	13%
w/8 oz 2% milk	8 oz	6	190	28%
w/8 oz whole milk	8 oz	8	280	26%
(Carnation) Slender/Can all flavors	10 oz	4	220	16%

BREAKFAST SANDWICH

Food and Description	Amount	Fat Grams	Total Calories	% Fat Calories
(Biscuits)				
(Hormel) New Traditions-frozen				
Egg, Bacon, & Cheese	1	13	280	42%
Ham & Egg	1	8	230	31%
Steak	1	15	330	41%
(Jimmy Dean) microwaveable				
Chicken	1	8	170	42%
Sausage	1	14	210	60%
Steak	1	11	190	52%
(Great Starts)				
Egg, Sausage & Cheese	1	28	460	55%
Sausage	1	22	410	48%
Muffins/(Healthy Choice)				
English Muffin Sandwich	1	3	200	14%
Turkey Sausage Omelet	1	4	210	17%
(Jimmy Dean) microwaveable				
Ham & cheese	1	4	130	28%
Sausage	1	11	190	52%
(Weight Watchers) Garden Vegetable Omelet/Ham & Cheese Bagel	1	6	210	26%

BROCCOLI DISHES

Food and Description	Amount	Fat Grams	Total Calories	% Fat Calories
Broccoli Crisp frozen (Ore Ida)	3 oz	11	190	52%
Broccoli in Cheese Sauce frozen (Birds Eye)	5 oz	6	120	45%

Food and Description	Amount	Fat Grams	Total Calories	% Fat Calories
Broccoli in White Cheddar Cheese Flavored Sauce				
frozen (Green Giant)	½ cup	3	50	54%
BROWNIES				
Box Mix/(Betty Crocker)				
Frosted (Stir'n Frost)	1	9	250	22%
Fudge (family size)	1	5	140	32%
(Betty Crocker) Microwave				
Frosted	1	7	180	35%
Fudge	1	6	150	36%
(Duncan Hines)				
Original Double Fudge	1	6	150	36%
Peanut Butter Fudge	1	8	150	48%
(Pillsbury)				
Deluxe Fudge Brownie	2" square	6	150	36%
Frozen/(Weight Watchers)				
Chocolate	1.25 oz	3	100	27%
Cheesecake	3.5 oz	5	200	23%
BUTTER				
sweet/salted and unsalted	1 pat	4	36	100%
BUTTER BLENDS				
(Blue Bonnet)/Stick and Tub	1 Tbs	11	90	100%
(Kraft) Touch of Butter Spread	1 Tbs	7	60	100%
BUTTER SUBSTITUTE				
Best of Butter/plain	½ tsp	< 1	4	100%
Butter Spray/(Weight Watchers)	1 spray	< 1	2	100%

C

Food and Description	Amount	Fat Grams	Total Calories	% Fat Calories
CAKE AND CAKE PASTRIES				
Apple Fruit Squares-frozen				
(Pepperidge Farm)	1	12	220	49%

Food and Description	Amount	Fat Grams	Total Calories	% Fat Calories
Banana-frozen (Sara Lee)	1 slice	6	170	32%
Black Forest-frozen (Sara Lee)	1 slice	8	190	38%
(Weight Watchers)	3 oz	5	180	25%
Boston Cream Pie frozen				
(Pepperidge Farm)	2⅞ oz	14	290	43%
(Weight Watchers)	3 oz	4	190	19%
Box mixes				
(Betty Crocker) Classics Dessert Mixes				
Boston Cream Pie	⅛ pkg	6	270	20%
Golden Pound Cake	1/12 cake	9	200	41%
Lemon Chiffon Cake	1/12 cake	4	200	18%
(Betty Crocker) Microwave box mixes w/frosting				
Choc Fudge w/van frost	⅙ cake	16	310	47%
Lemon w/lemon frosting	⅙ cake	16	300	48%
Pineapple Upside-Down	⅑ cake	10	250	36%
(Betty Crocker) Supermoist				
Butter Recipe/chocolate	1/12 cake	13	270	43%
Chocolate Chip	1/12 cake	14	280	45%
Yellow	1/12 cake	11	260	38%
(Betty Crocker) Supermoist Light Mixes				
Devils Food/No Cholesterol	1/12 cake	3	180	15%
Standard Recipe	1/12 cake	4	190	19%
(Duncan Hines) Delights				
Devil's Food	1/12 cake	5	180	25%
Yellow	1/12 cake	4	180	20%
(Duncan Hines) Original Directions				
Butter Recipe/Fudge	1/12 cake	13	270	43%
Swiss Chocolate	1/12 cake	15	280	48%
Yellow	1/12 cake	11	260	38%
(Pillsbury) Bundt Brand Ring				
Pound	1/16 cake	9	230	35%
(Pillsbury) Microwave box mixes				
Chocolate Cake	⅛ cake	13	210	56%
Yellow	⅛ cake	13	220	53%
Cheesecake (9" dia)	1/12 cake	18	280	58%
Frozen/(Sara Lee) French	1 slice	13	200	59%
(Weight Watchers)				
Cherries & Cream	3 oz	2	130	14%

Food and Description	Amount	Fat Grams	Total Calories	% Fat Calories
Chocolate/(Pepperidge Farm)	2⅞ oz	17	310	49%
(Weight Watchers)	2.5 oz	5	180	25%
Cinnamon bun/plain	1/~ 2 oz	5	174	26%
refrig w/icing (Pillsbury)	1	4.5	115	35%
Coffeecake				
(Pillsbury) Apple Cinnamon	⅛ cake	7	240	26%
(Hostess) 97% fat free				
Cinnamon Crumb Cake	1 cake	1	80	11%
(Sara Lee) frozen				
Apple Cinnamon	1 cake	13	290	40%
Pecan	1 cake	16	280	51%
(Weight Watcher) frozen				
Streusel w/cinnamon	2.25 oz	7	190	33%
(Entenmann's) Regular Bakery Line				
All Butter Pound	1 oz	5	110	41%
Cheese Coffee Cake	1.6 oz	7	150	42%
Thick Fudge Golden Cake	1.2 oz	6	130	42%
Fruit Squares-frozen				
(Pepperidge Farm)/Apple	1	12	220	49%
German Chocolate				
(Pepperidge Farm)	1⅝ oz	10	180	50%
(Weight Watchers)	2.5 oz	7	200	32%
(Pepperidge Farm) Dessert Light-individual servings-frozen				
Apple'n Spice	1 pkg	2	170	11%
Strawberry ShortCake	1 pkg	5	170	27%
(Sara Lee) Lights-frozen				
Chocolate Mousse	1 pkg	9	180	45%
Strawberry Cheese Cake	1 pkg	4	160	23%
Strawberry Short Cake-frozen				
(Sara Lee)	1 slice	8	190	38%
(Weight Watchers)	3 oz	4	160	23%
Turnovers/frozen				
(Pepperidge Farm)/Apple	1	17	300	51%
(Pillsbury) /refrige-.All flavors	1	8	170	42%
Vanilla-frozen (Pepperidge Farm)	1⅝ oz	8	190	38%
CANDY				
Almond Joy (Peter Paul)	1.76 oz	14	250	50%
Alpine w/almonds	1.3 oz	13	200	59%

Food and Description	Amount	Fat Grams	Total Calories	% Fat Calories
Butterscotch	1 oz	1	113	8%
Carmello (Cadbury's)	1 oz	7	140	45%
Cherries-chocolate covered	1	3	90	30%
Chocolate				
Special Dark (Hershey)	1 bar	12	220	49%
Chunky-milk chocolate	1 oz	4	120	30%
original	1 oz	7	143	44%
Good & Plenty	1 oz	< 1	106	4%
Junior Mints	1 oz	3	120	23%
Kisses (Hershey's) plain	1 kiss	1	25	36%
Kit Kat	1.5 oz	12	230	47%
M & M's/Almond	1.3 oz	10	200	45%
Peanut	1.6 oz	12	240	45%
Plain	1 oz	6	140	39%
Malt Balls-chocolate covered	2 pieces	4	50	72%
Milk Chocolate Bar/(Hershey)	1.55 oz	14	240	53%
w/almonds	1.45 oz	14	230	55%
Milk Duds	1 oz	4	129	28%
Milky Way (Mars)	3.63 oz	18	470	35%
Dark	1.76 oz	8	220	33%
Mounds Bar (Hershey)	1.9 oz	14	260	48%
Peppermint Patties/(York)	1 oz	3	120	23%
Raisinets (Nestle)	1.6 oz	7	200	32%
Reese's Peanut Butter Cups	2 cups	18	200	81%
Reese's Pieces (Hershey)	1.95 pkg	11	270	37%
Snickers (Mars)/plain	2.07 oz	14	280	45%
3 Musketeers	1 oz	4	120	30%
Tootsie Roll	1 large	2.6	127	18%
Twix Caramel	2 oz	14	280	45%
Twizzlers-Strawberry (Y&S)	1 oz	< 1	100	5%
CAULIFLOWER DISHES				
in butter sauce (Green Giant)	½ cup	1	30	30%
in cheese flav. (Green Giant)	½ cup	2	60	30%

CEREAL (NOTE: All cereals are either dry or prepared with water per directions on packaging. If milk is used, calorie and fat content increase accordingly. Data on milk is shown in the Quick Reference on the next page. For additional information on milk, see MILK.)

Food and Description	Amount	Fat Grams	Total Calories	% Fat Calories

QUICK REFERENCE: MILK

Food and Description	Amount	Fat Grams	Total Calories	% Fat Calories
Skim	¼ cup	–	23	–
	½ cup	–	45	–
1% lowfat	¼ cup	.5	26	17%
	½ cup	1	55	16%
2% lowfat	¼ cup	1	31	29%
	½ cup	2.5	61	37%
Whole	¼ cup	2	38	47%
	½ cup	4	75	48%

Food and Description	Amount	Fat Grams	Total Calories	% Fat Calories
■ HOT/COOKED CEREAL				
Bran (Health Valley)/100% Natural Bran Cereal				
w/raisins	¼ cup	1	100	9%
100% Organic w/raisins	1 oz	< 1	90	5%
Farina/Dry	1 cup	1	649	1%
Oat Bran/(Arrowhead Mills)	1 serving	2	110	16%
(Health Valley) 100% natural-hot				
Apple Cinnamon	1 serving	1	100	9%
(Nabisco) Wholesome'N Hearty	1 serving	2	90	20%
Oatmeal, Instant (General Mills)				
Apple cinnamon/raspberry	1 package	2	160	11%
(Quaker)/Extra-fortified Instant				
Raisins & Cinnamon	1 package	2	130	17%
Regular	1 package	2	100	18%
Whole Wheat Hot Natural Cereal				
(Quaker's)	1 serving	1	90	10%
■ COLD/READY-TO-EAT CEREAL				
Alpen Muesli Raisins & Nuts	½ cup	3	220	12%
Alpha-Bits (Post)	1 cup	1	110	6%
Basic 4 (General Mills)	¾ cup	2	130	14%
Bran (*See also* Oat Bran, in this listing)				
All Bran (Kellogg's)/Original	⅓ cup	1	70	13%
Fruit & almonds	⅓ cup	2	100	18%
Bran Chex	⅔ cup	.7	90	7%
Fruitful Bran (Kellogg's)	⅔ cup	1	120	8%

Food and Description	Amount	Fat Grams	Total Calories	% Fat Calories
Mueslix	½ cup	2	140	13%
Cap'n Crunch	¾ cup	2	110	16%
Cheerios, Original	¾ cup	2	110	16%
Apple Cinnamon	¾ cup	2	110	16%
Honey Nut	¾ cup	1	110	8%
Cocoa Puffs (General Mills)	1 oz/1 cup	1	110	8%
✴ Corn Flakes (Kellogg's)	1 cup	0	100	0
Count Chocula (General Mills)	1 cup	1	110	8%
Cracklin Oat Bran (Kellogg's)	½ cup	3	110	25%
Froot Loops (Kellogg's)	1 oz/1 cup	1	110	8%
✦ Frosted Krispies (Kellogg's)	⅔ cup	1	110	8%
Fruit & Fibre (Post)				
Dates/raisins/walnuts	⅔ cup	2	120	15%
Golden Grahams	¾ cup	1	110	8%
Life (Quaker)/Cinnamon	⅔ cup	1.6	110	13%
Lucky Charms (General Mills)	1 cup	1	110	8%
Nut & Honey Crunch (Kellogg's)	⅔ cup	1	110	8%
Oat Chex (Ralston)	1 oz	1	100	9%
Shredded Wheat/(Nabisco)				
Original	1 biscuit	1	80	11%
(Quaker) Original	2 biscuits	1	130	7%
Teenage Mutant Ninja Turtles	1 oz	1	110	8%
Total (General Mills)/Corn Flakes	1 cup	< 1	110	4%
Raisin Bran	1.5 oz	1	140	6%
Trix (General Mills)	1.5 oz	1	119	8%
Wheaties (General Mills)	1 cup	1	100	9%
CHEESE				
American/(Alpine Lace)	1 oz	6	80	67%
(Borden) Processed Slices	1 oz	9	110	74%
Light 15% Milkfat	1 oz	5	70	64%
Singles	1 oz	7	90	70%
(Land O'Lakes) Processed	1 oz	9	110	74%
Swiss-Processed	1 oz	8	100	72%
(Lite-Line)	⅔ oz	2	35	51%
(Weight Watchers)	1 oz	2	50	36%
American-Swiss/(Formagg)	¾ oz	5	70	64%
(Land O'Lakes)	1 oz	9	100	81%
Blue	1 oz	8	100	72%

Food and Description	Amount	Fat Grams	Total Calories	% Fat Calories
(Kraft)	1 oz	9	100	81%
Brick	1 oz	9	110	74%
Natural (Land O'Lakes)	1 oz	8	110	66%
Snack-Pasteurized Process	1 oz	9	100	81%
Brie	1 oz	7.85	95	74%
(Fromageries Bel)	1 oz	8	90	80%
Cheddar/(Alpine Lace)	1 oz	5	80	56%
Extra Sharp (Land O'Lakes)				
Process	1 oz	9	100	81%
Imitation (Sargento)	1 oz	6	90	60%
(Weight Watchers)				
Shredded-Part Skim Milk	1 oz	5	80	56%
Mild	1 oz	9	114	71%
(Kraft) Healthy Favorites-				
Shredded	1 oz	4	70	51%
(Sargento)	1 oz	9	110	74%
(Weight Watchers)	1 oz	5	80	56%
Natural/(Cracker Barrel) Light				
Reduced Fat Sharp-White	1 oz	5	80	53%
(Kraft)	1 oz	9	110	74%
Light Naturals Reduced Fat	1 oz	5	80	56%
(Weight Watchers)	1 oz	5	80	56%
Sharp/(Light N'Lively)	1 oz	4	70	51%
(Lite-Line) 8% Milkfat	1 oz	2	50	36%
(Sargento) Nut Log	1 oz	7	100	63%
(Weight Watchers)	1 oz	2	50	36%
Singles-Cheese Food/(Kraft)	1 oz	8	100	72%
Cheese Sauce /Canned	2 oz	4	60	60%
Mix	4 oz	18	225	72%
Nacho (Kaukauna)	1 oz	6	80	68%
Cheese Spreads				
American Pasteurized (Kraft)	1 oz	6	80	68%
American Sharp Pasteurized Processed				
(Sargento)	1 oz	9	110	74%
(Cheez Whiz) Plain	1 oz	5.7	80	64%
Country Crock (Shedds)				
Fresh Cheddar	1 oz	4	70	51%
Fresh Garden Vegetable	1 oz	7	70	90%

Food and Description	Amount	Fat Grams	Total Calories	% Fat Calories
Jalapeno Pasteurized-Loaf	1 oz	6	80	68%
Pimiento (Kraft)	1 oz	5	70	64%
Spreadery (Kraft) Cheese Snack				
Medium Cheddar Cold Pack	1 oz	4	70	51%
Velveeta Spread (Kraft)/Light	1 oz	4	70	51%
Original	1 oz	6	80	68%
Slices	1 oz	6	90	60%
Cheese & Sticks (Sargento)	1 oz	6	110	49%
(Cracker Barrel) Cheese Ball				
Sharp Cheddar w/Almonds	1 oz	7	100	63%
Cream Cheese	1 oz	9.89	99	90%
✳ (Philadelphia Brand)				
Light Pasteurized Process	1 oz	5	60	75%
Soft/Original	1 oz	10	100	90%
(Weight Watchers)	1 oz	2	35	51%
Feta/(Sargento)	1 oz	6	80	68%
Gouda/(Kraft)-Natural	1 oz	9	110	74%
Italian Style Grated Cheeses				
(Sargento)	1 oz	8	110	66%
Limburger	1 oz	7.7	93	75%
Monterey	1 oz	8.58	106	73%
Monterey Jack/(Alpine Lace)	1 oz	5	80	56%
(Kraft)/Cheese Food Singles	1 oz	7	90	70%
Mozzarella				
Imitation (Sargento)	1 oz	6	80	68%
(Lite-Line) 8% Milkfat				
Pasteurized Process	1 oz	2	50	36%
Natural (Kraft) Light Naturals				
Healthy Favorites-Shredded	1 oz	3	60	45%
(Weight Watchers)	1 oz	4	70	51%
Part Skim (Alpine Lace)	1 oz	5	70	64%
Muenster (Alpine Lace)	1 oz	9	100	81%
(Kraft)	1 oz	9	110	74%
Nacho (Sargento)	1 oz	9	106	76%
Nacho Cheese Dip/(Kraft)	2 Tbs	4	50	72%
Parmesan/Fresh				
✳ (Sargento)/Grated	1 Tbs	1.5	23	59%
Hard	1 oz	7	111	57%

Food and Description	Amount	Fat Grams	Total Calories	% Fat Calories
Pizza Double Cheese (Sargento)				
Light Shredded	1 oz	4	70	51%
Pizza Topper (Formagg)	1 oz	5	70	64%
Port Wine Nut Log (Sargento)	1 oz	7	100	63%
Provolone/(Alpine Lace)	1 oz	5	70	64%
(Sargento)	1 oz	8	100	72%
Ricotta/(Sargento)/Lite	1 oz	1	25	36%
Part Skim	1 oz	2	30	60%
Whole Milk/Generic	½ cup	16	216	67%
Romano (Kraft)/ grated	1 oz	9	130	62%
String Cheese (Sargento)/Plain	1 oz	5	80	56%
Swiss/Aged (Kraft)	1 oz	8	110	66%
Almond Nut Log (Sargento)	1 oz	7	90	70%
(Alpine Lace) Swiss-Lo	1 oz	6	90	60%
(Cracker Barrel) Natural Babys	1 oz	9	110	65%
(Kraft)/Deluxe Slices	1 oz	7	90	70%
(Sargento)/Natural	1 oz	8	110	66%
Snack-Pasteurized Process	1 oz	7	100	63%
(Weight Watchers)	1 oz	2	50	36%
Natural	1 oz	5	80	56%
Taco-(Kraft)/Shredded	1 oz	9	110	74%
CHEESE SUBSTITUTE				
(Delica)/ American pasteurized				
process	1 oz	6	80	68%
(Formagg) no lactose - lower in saturated fat - made w/canola oil				
American/white	1 oz	5	70	64%
Ricotta	1 oz	.85	35	22%
CHICKEN				
Chicken, broilers, or fryers-flesh only				
fried	~ 5 oz	12.77	307	37%
roasted w/skin	~ 5 oz	10	266	34%
stewed w/skin	~ 5 oz	9	248	33%
Chicken-Light Meat w/skin				
batter dipped/fried	~ 7 oz	29	520	50%
roasted	~ 5 oz	14	293	43%
Chicken-Light Meat w/o skin				
fried	~ 5 oz	7.76	268	26%
roasted	~ 5 oz	6	242	22%

Food and Description	Amount	Fat Grams	Total Calories	% Fat Calories
stewed	~ 5 oz	5.58	223	23%
Chicken Breast/meat & skin				
batter dipped/fried	~ 5 oz	18.5	364	46%
roasted	~ 3.5 oz	7.6	193	35%
Chicken Breast/meat only				
fried	~ 3 oz	4	161	22%
roasted	~ 3 oz	3	142	19%
stewed	~ 3 oz	2.88	144	18%
Chicken Leg/meat & skin				
batter dipped/fried	~ 5.5 oz	25.55	431	53%
flour coated/fried	~ 4 oz	16	285	51%
roasted	~ 4 oz	15	265	51%
stewed	~ 4 oz	16	275	52%
Chicken Leg/meat only				
fried	~ 3 oz	8.76	195	40%
roasted	~ 3 oz	8	182	40%
stewed	~ 3.5 oz	8	187	39%
Chicken Thigh/meat & skin				
batter dipped/fried	~ 3 oz	14	238	53%
flour coated/fried	~ 2 oz	9	162	50%
roasted	~ 2 oz	9.6	153	56%
stewed	~ 2 oz	10	158	57%
Chicken Thigh/meat only				
fried	~ 2 oz	5	113	40%
roasted	~ 2 oz	5.66	109	47%
stewed	~ 2 oz	5	107	42%
Chicken, Roasting/roasted				
meat & skin	~ 5 oz	9	233	35%
light meat/meat only	~ 5 oz	5.7	214	34%
(Perdue)				
Cornish Game Hen/fresh-after roasting 1-oz uncooked portion				
dark meat w/skin	1 oz	3.3	49	61%
white meat w/skin	1 oz	2.3	41	50%
Oven Stuffer Roaster/fresh-after roasting 1-oz uncooked portion				
breast/boneless	1 oz	.3	28	10%
whole	1 oz	2	40	45%
dark meat w/skin	1 oz	3.1	46	61%
drumsticks	1 oz	2.1	40	47%

Food and Description	Amount	Fat Grams	Total Calories	% Fat Calories
thigh/boneless cutlets	1 oz	1.9	37	46%
whole	1 oz	3.5	50	63%
white meat w/skin	1 oz	2.2	42	47%
CHICKEN ENTREE/DINNER				
Chicken and Rice/box-mixes prepared				
Almond Chicken-Wild Rice				
(Savory Classics)	1 serving	4	140	26%
Chicken-Broccoli-Dijon				
(Savory Classics)	1 serving	5	160	28%
Chicken Flavor (Rice-A-Roni)	1 serving	1	130	7%
Chicken & Vegetables				
(Rice-A-Roni)	1 serving	3	140	19%
Chicken-Vermicelli				
(Rice-A-Roni)	1 serving	5	170	27%
Chicken Cacciatore				
(Lean Cuisine) frozen	~ 11 oz	10	280	32%
Chicken Pot Pies/Frozen				
(Morton)	7 oz	28	420	60%
(Swanson)	7 oz	22	380	52%
(Swanson) frozen Plump & Juicy Chicken				
Chicken Nuggets	8¾ oz	25	460	49%
Fried Chicken-breast portion	4½ oz	22	360	55%
(Weaver)/Frozen Boneless Portions				
Batter Dipped/Assorted	3.6 oz	18	290	56%
Chicken Nuggets	2.6 oz	12	190	57%
Hot Wings	2.7 oz	11	170	48%
CHICKEN SEASONING				
(French's) Microwave Mixes				
Barbecue Chicken	¼ pkg	2	50	36%
(Lipton) Microeasy Family Favorites - dry				
Barbeque Style Chicken	¼ pkg	.5	108	4%
Country Style Chicken	¼ pkg	.6	78	7%
CHOCOLATE, BAKING				
(Baker's)/Semi-sweet bar	1 oz	9	140	58%
Unsweetened	1 oz	15	140	96%
(Hershey's)/Premium bar				
Semi-sweet	1 oz	8	140	51%
Unsweetened	1 oz	16	190	76%

Food and Description	Amount	Fat Grams	Total Calories	% Fat Calories
(Nestles)/Pre-melted-Unsweetened				
Choco Bake	1 oz	16	190	76%
Premier white	1 oz	5	80	56%
Semi-sweet	1 oz	9	160	51%
Unsweetened	1 oz	14	180	70%
CHOCOLATE CHIPS & CHUNKS				
(Baker's)/Milk chocolate	1 oz	8	140	51%
Semi-sweet/Big chips	¼ cup	13	220	53%
Flavored	½ cup	18	380	43%
(Hershey's)/Milk chocolate				
Chips	1 oz	8	150	48%
Mint	¼ cup	12	230	47%
Semi-sweet/Chips	¼ cup	12	220	49%
(Nestles)/Butterscotch	1 oz	8	150	48%
Chocolate	1 oz	7	150	42%
Semi-sweet	1 oz	8	150	48%
CLAM				
breaded & fried	3 oz	9	171	47%
steamed	3 oz	1.65	126	12%
COCOA				
(Baker's)	3.5 oz	13	220	53%
(Hershey's)/Original	⅓ cup	3	110	25%
(Nestles)	½ cup	6	180	30%
COCONUT				
(Baker's) Angel Flake/Package	⅓ cup	8	120	60%
Toasted	⅓ cup	17	200	77%
(Durkee) Shredded	1 cup	28	277	91%
COCONUT CREAM				
Canned, sweetened	1 Tbs	3	36	75%
(Coco Lopez)	2 Tbs	5	120	38%
COOKIE				
Animal (Sunshine)	14 cookies	3	120	23%
Chocolate Chip/box mix				
(Duncan Hines)	2 cookies	5	130	35%
(Entenmann's)	3 cookies	7	130	48%
refrigerated dough (2¼" dia)	4 cookies	11	225	44%
(Famous Amos)/Chocolate Chip-no nuts				
Chocolate Chip w/Pecans	1 oz	8	151	48%

Food and Description	Amount	Fat Grams	Total Calories	% Fat Calories
Oatmeal w/Cinnamon & Raisins	1 oz	6	133	41%
Fig Bars	4 bars	4	210	17%
(Keebler)/Chips Deluxe	1 cookie	4	80	45%
Deluxe Grahams-Fudge Cover	1 cookie	2	40	45%
E.L. Fudge Sandwich	1 cookie	3	70	39%
Pecan Sandies	1 cookie	5	80	56%
Oatmeal Cremes	1 cookie	3	80	34%
Soft Batch/Chocolate Chip	1 cookie	4	80	45%
Vanilla Wafers	5 cookies	5	100	45%
(Nabisco)/Almost Home				
Fudge Chocolate Chip	1 cookie	3	70	39%
Oatmeal Raisin	1 cookie	3	70	39%
Chips Ahoy				
Chewy Chocolate Chip	1 cookie	3	60	45%
Mini Chocolate Chip	6 cookies	3	70	39%
Devil's Food Cakes	1 cake	1	70	13%
Famous Cookie Assortment				
Baronet Creme Sandwich	3 cookies	6	140	39%
Biscos Sugar Wafers	3 wafers	7	150	42%
Butter-Flavored	6 cookies	5	130	35%
Cameo Creme Sandwich	2 cookies	5	140	31%
Lorna Doone Shortbread	4 cookies	7	140	45%
Mallomars Chocolate Cakes	1 piece	3	60	45%
Newtons Fruit Chewy Cookies				
Apple	1 cookie	2	70	26%
Fig Newtons	1 cookie	1	60	15%
Variety Pack/all flavors	1 cookie	3	120	23%
Nilla Wafers/Original	3½ cookie	2	60	30%
Old Fashion Ginger Snaps	1 cookie	1	30	30%
Oreo Double Stuf Chocolate	1 cookie	4	70	51%
Oatmeal Chocolate Chip	1 cookie	3	60	45%
Oatmeal w/raisins	4 cookies	10	245	37%
box mix (Duncan Hines)	2 cookies	6	130	42%
packaged/(Duncan Hines)	2 cookies	5	110	41%
(Pepperidge Farm) American Collection Cookies				
Beacon Hill Brownie Nut	1 cookie	7	120	52%
Chesapeake Chocolate Chunk Pecan	1 cookie	7	120	53%

Food and Description	Amount	Fat Grams	Total Calories	% Fat Calories
Nantucket Chocolate Chunk	1 cookie	6	120	45%
Sante Fe Oatmeal Raisin	1 cookie	4	100	36%
Distinctive Cookies/Linzer	1 cookie	4	120	30%
Milano	2 cookies	6	120	45%
(Stella D'Oro)/Anisette Toast	1 cookie	.6	46	12%
Breakfast Treats	1 piece	3.6	101	32%
Coconut Macaroons	1 cookie	3	60	45%
Sesame, Dietetic	1 piece	2	43	42%
(Sunshine)/Butter Flavored	2 cookies	2	60	30%
Fig Bars	2 cookies	2	90	20%
Hydrox/Original	1 cookie	2	50	36%
Vanilla Wafers	6 wafers	6	130	42%
CORN				
Sweet-white or yellow/cooked	½ cup	1	89	10%
Canned/(Green Giant)	½ cup	1	100	9%
Frozen/Cob Corn (Ore Ida)	1 ear	1	150	6%
cream style	½ cup	.6	120	5%
cut (Pictsweet)	3.2 oz	1	80	11%
CORNED BEEF				
Brisket	3 oz	16	213	68%
Canned (Hormel) 12 oz	2 oz	8	130	55%
CORNED BEEF HASH				
(Armour) Premium Lite	7.5 oz	21	350	54%
Original	7.5 oz	27	390	62%
COTTAGE CHEESE				
(Light N' Lively)	4 oz	1	80	11%
2% lowfat	4 oz	2	101	18%
(Weight Watchers)/1%	4 oz	1	90	10%
CRACKER CRUMBS-GRAHAM				
(Nabisco)/Original	2 Tbs	1	60	15%
(Sunshine)	½ cup	7	275	23%
CRACKERS				
Cheese (Ritz)	10	6	140	39%
Cheese & Peanut Butter (Ritz)	6	10	210	43%
Chowder and Oyster (O.T.C.)	1	1	25	36%
(Eagle) Snack Crackers/Cheese	1 oz	6	130	42%
Graham Crackers/(Honey Maid) Cinnamon	2	1	60	15%

Food and Description	Amount	Fat Grams	Total Calories	% Fat Calories
Plain	2	1	60	15%
(Keebler)/Cinnamon Crisp	1	2	70	26%
Honey Grahams	4	3	80	34%
(Nabisco)	2	1	60	15%
(Sunshine) Cinnamon	1	3	70	39%
Hi-Ho (Sunshine)/Original Deluxe	4	5	80	56%
(Keebler)/Cheddar Cracker Chips	18	3	70	39%
Club/Original & Low Salt	4	3	60	45%
Whole Wheat	4	3	70	39%
Town House	5	5	80	56%
(Nabisco)/Cheese Tid-Bits	16	4	70	51%
Chocolate Grahams	1 piece	3	60	45%
Garden Crisps/Vegetable	7 pieces	2	60	30%
Premium Saltine	5	2	60	30%
Ritz/Regular & Low-Salt	4	4	70	51%
Whole Wheat	5	2	60	30%
Sociable	6	3	70	39%
Swiss Cheese Snack	7½	3	70	39%
Triscuit Wafers/Wheat'n Bran	3	2	60	30%
Vegetable Thins	6	4	70	51%
Wheat Thins/Cheese	8	3	70	39%
Zwieback Teething Toast	2 pieces	1	60	15%
(Sunshine)/Cheez-it	12	4	70	51%
Whole Wheat (Manischewitz)	10	1	90	10%
CREAM				
Coffee/Table light cream	1 Tbs	3	30	90%
Coffee Lightener-non-dairy/frozen				
(Carnation) Coffee Mate	1 Tbs	1	16	56%
(Half & Half)	1 Tbs	1.7	20	77%
(Cremora) Original	1 tsp	1	12	75%
Whipping Cream heavy	1 cup	88	820	100%
CROUTON				
(Pepperidge Farm)				
Cheddar & Romano Cheese	½ oz	2	60	30%
(Progresso) Italian Style	½ oz	1	30	30%

D

Food and Description	Amount	Fat Grams	Total Calories	% Fat Calories
DIPS				
(Hain)/Mexican Bean	2 Tbs	1	35	23%
(Kraft)/Avocado (Guacamole)	2 Tbs	4	50	72%
French Onion	2 Tbs	4	60	60%
Premium Nacho Cheese	2 Tbs	4	55	65%
(Slender Choice)/French Onion	1 Tbs	1	14	64%
Jalapeno	1 Tbs	1	16	56%
DONUT				
(Drake's)/Old Fashioned	1 pkg	8	180	40%
Powdered Sugar	1 pkg	15	300	45%
(Entenmann's)/Crumb Topped	1	12	260	42%
Devil's Food	1	12	250	43%
Rich Frosted	1	18	280	58%
(Hostess) Breakfast Bake Shop				
Cinnamon 8 Pack	1	6	140	39%
Pantry (assorted)	1	10	190	47%
Crumb/Frosted &/or Plain	1	5	80	56%
Donut Gems, Plain	1	3	60	45%
Old Fashioned/Glazed	1	12	250	43%
Plain	1	9	170	48%
Powdered Sugar/8 Pack	1	7	140	45%
Pantry (assorted)	1	10	190	47%
(Little Debbie)/Donut Sticks	2.5 oz	18	330	49%
(Tastykake)/Assorted (9 count)				
Cinnamon	1	8	180	40%
Plain	1	10	190	47%
Mini/Cinnamon	1	2	50	36%
Powdered Sugar	1	1	40	23%
DUCK				
Domestic				
Meat & Skin-roasted	12 oz	108	1287	76%
Meat only-roasted	8 oz	25	445	50%

E

Food and Description	Amount	Fat Grams	Total Calories	% Fat Calories
EGG/Chicken-large/boiled	1 egg	5.6	79	64%
EGG MEALS				
Deviled	1 egg	13	145	81%
Scrambled Eggs/Frozen				
(Aunt Jemima)/& Sausage				
w/Hash Browns	5.7 oz	20	290	62%
w/Pancakes	5.2 oz	14	270	47%
(Downyflake)				
w/Ham & Hash Browns	6¼ oz	26	350	67%
(Swanson-Great Starts)				
w/Bacon & Home Fries	5¼ oz	26	340	69%
EGGNOG				
Canned/(Borden)	4 oz	9	160	51%
Commercial/(Carnation) Lite	8 oz	8	320	23%
(Kemps)/Original	4 oz	9	175	46%
(Land O'Lakes)/Original	8 oz	7	380	17%
EGGPLANT DISHES				
Eggplant Parmigiana/frozen				
(Celantano)	8 oz	15	280	48%
(Mrs. Paul's)	5 oz	16	240	60%

F

Food and Description	Amount	Fat Grams	Total Calories	% Fat Calories
FIG				
(Sun Maid)/Calimyma	½ cup	2	250	7%

Food and Description	Amount	Fat Grams	Total Calories	% Fat Calories
Mission	½ cup	1	210	4%
FLOUNDER				
baked w/butter	3 oz	7	171	37%
baked w/o butter	3 oz	1	80	11%
frozen-breaded	5 oz	15	300	45%
frozen-raw (Van de Kamp's)	4 oz	1	100	9%
FLOUR				
Amaranth	1 cup	2	698	3%
Barley	1 Tbs	< 1	28	16%
Bread/(Gold Medal) high protein	1 cup	1	400	2%
(Pillsbury's Best)	1 cup	2	400	5%
Brown Rice	2 oz	1	200	5%
Cake or Pastry	4 oz	1	413	2%
Corn	1 cup	3	430	6%
Cracked Wheat (Krusteaz)	1 cup	2	320	6%
Oat (Arrowhead Mills)	2 oz	1	200	5%
Oat Flour Blend (Gold Medal)	4 oz	3	390	7%
Rye, (Pillsbury)	1 cup	2	400	5%
Soybean, low-fat	1 cup	6	326	17%
White, all purpose	1 cup	1	401	2%
Whole Wheat	1 cup	2	400	5%
FRANKFURTER				
(Ball Park)				
Lite	1	12	140	77%
Weiners, Beef	1	16	175	82%
(Butterball) Turkey	1	11	130	76%
(Hebrew National) Beef	1.7 oz	14	150	84%
(Hormel) Beef	1	13	140	84%
(Kahn's) Beef Jumbo	2 oz	16	190	76%
(Oscar Meyer) Beef Franks	2 oz	17	180	85%
(Perdue) Chicken	1 oz	5.7	71	72%
(Tyson) Cheese Franks	1	11	145	68%
(Weaver) Chicken Cheese	1	11	145	68%
FRENCH TOAST				
Frozen (Aunt Jemima)/Original	2 slices	4	166	22%
Sticks w/Syrup	5.2 oz	20	400	45%
(Downyflake)/Cinnamon	2 slices	7	210	30%
Plain	2 slices	12	270	40%

Food and Description	Amount	Fat Grams	Total Calories	% Fat Calories
(Weight Watchers) Cinnamon	3 oz	4	160	23%
FROZEN DAIRY DESSERT				
(Dreyer's)/Frozen Dietary Dessert				
Chocolate	4 oz	7	140	45%
Vanilla	4 oz	7	130	49%
(Edy's)/Chocolate	½ cup	7	140	45%
Vanilla	½ cup	7	130	49%
(Healthy Choice)/Chocolate	4 oz	2	130	14%
Cookies'N Cream	4 oz	2	130	14%
Rocky Road	4 oz	2	160	11%
Vanilla	4 oz	2	120	15%
(Simplesse) Simple Pleasures				
Chocolate	½ cup	< 1	140	3%
Chocolate Chip	½ cup	3	150	18%
Mint Chocolate Chip	½ cup	2	150	12%
Vanilla	½ cup	< 1	120	4%
(Sweet'N Low)/Chocolate	4 oz	2	90	20%
Strawberry	4 oz	1	80	11%
Vanilla	4 oz	2	80	23%
FROZEN ENTREE/DINNER				
(Banquet)/Entree Express				
Extra Helping Dinners/Beef	15.5 oz	13	430	27%
Fried Chicken	14.25 oz	43	790	49%
Turkey	17 oz	12	460	23%
Family Entrees/Beef Stew	7 oz	5	140	32%
Chicken Primavera	7 oz	3	140	19%
Gravy & Salisbury Steak	7 oz	19	260	66%
Gravy & Sliced Turkey	6 oz	6	120	45%
(Budget Gourmet)/Light & Healthy Dinners				
Chicken Breast Parmigiana	11 oz	8	260	28%
Sirloin Salisbury Steak	11 oz	9	260	31%
Teriyaki Chicken Breast	11 oz	6	270	20%
Light & Healthy Dinners				
Herbed Chicken	11 oz	7	240	26%
Special Recipe Sirloin Beef	11 oz	10	250	36%
Stuffed Turkey Breast	11 oz	6	230	23%
(Celentano) Entrees				
Broccoli Stuffed Shells	6.75 oz	14	270	47%

Food and Description	Amount	Fat Grams	Total Calories	% Fat Calories
Eggplant Parmigiana	10 oz	19	350	49%
Lasagna Primavera	11 oz	14	330	38%
Ravioli	6.5 oz	11	380	26%
(Healthy Choice) Dinners				
Beef Pepper Steak	11 oz	6	290	19%
Breast of Turkey	10.5 oz	5	290	16%
Pasta Primavera	11 oz	3	280	10%
Salsa Chicken	11.25 oz	2	240	8%
Shrimp Marinara	10.5 oz	1	260	3%
Sweet & Sour Chicken	11.5 oz	2	280	6%
Teriyaki Chicken	12.25 oz	4	290	12%
Entrees/Beef Pepper Steak	9.5 oz	4	250	14%
Cheese Manicotti	9.25 oz	3	220	12%
Chicken & Vegetables	11.5 oz	1	210	4%
Lasagna w/meat sauce	10 oz	5	260	17%
Linguini w/Shrimp	9.5 oz	2	230	8%
Seafood Newburg	8 oz	3	200	14%
Lean Cuisine (Stouffer's)				
Breast of Chicken Marsala	8⅛ oz	5	190	24%
Broccoli & Cheddar Potato	10⅜ oz	9	290	28%
Chicken & Vegetables	11¾ oz	6	250	22%
Chicken Cacciatore	10⅞ oz	7	280	23%
Chicken Chow Mein w/Rice	9 oz	5	240	19%
Filet of Fish Divan	10⅜ oz	5	210	21%
Lasagna w/Meat Sauce	10¼ oz	6	260	21%
Macaroni & Cheese	9 oz	9	290	28%
Sliced Turkey Breast	7⅞ oz	5	200	23%
(Stouffer's)/Entrees				
Beef Stroganoff w/ Noodles	9.75 oz	20	390	46%
Chicken Divan	8.5 oz	20	320	56%
Lasagna, Single Serving	10.5 oz	13	360	33%
Macaroni & Cheese (12 oz)	6 oz	13	250	47%
Vegetable Lasagna	10.5 oz	24	420	51%
Hungry Man Dinners				
Fried Chicken, White Meat	14.25 oz	46	870	48%
Salisbury Steak	18.25 oz	41	680	54%
Turkey	17 oz	18	550	30%
Veal Parmigiana	18.25 oz	26	590	40%

Food and Description	Amount	Fat Grams	Total Calories	% Fat Calories
(Tyson) /Healthy Portion Meals				
BBQ Chicken Meal	12.5 oz	8	470	15%
Chicken Marinara	13.75 oz	7	330	19%
Sesame Chicken	13.5 oz	5	390	12%
(Weight Watchers)/Entrees				
Angel Hair Pasta	10 oz	4	200	18%
Baked Cheese Ravioli	9 oz	6	240	23%
Baked Potatoe/Broc & Cheese	10.5 oz	6	270	20%
Beef Stroganoff	8.5 oz	9	280	29%
Chicken Divan Potato	11.25 oz	7	280	23%
Stuffed Turkey Breast	8.5 oz	8	270	27%
FRUIT SNACKS				
(Del Monte)/Sierra Trail Mix	.9 oz	7	130	49%
Tropical Fruit Punch	.9 oz	1	90	10%
Yogurt Raisins	.9 oz	< 1	120	38%

G

Food and Description	Amount	Fat Grams	Total Calories	% Fat Calories
GEFILTE FISH				
(Manischewitz)/sweet	3.5 oz	4	132	27%
GELATIN				
(Jell-O) 1-2-3/Strawberry	⅔ cup	2	130	14%
GRANOLA/GRANOLA-TYPE BARS				
(Health Valley) Bakes/Apple	1 bar	3	100	27%
Fat-Free Fruit/Apple	1 bar	< 1	140	3%
Fat-Free Granola/Date Almond	1 bar	< 1	140	3%
Raisin Cinnamon	1 oz	< 1	90	5%
Fruit & Fitness Bars	2 bars	5	200	23%
(Kudos)/Chocolate Chip	1 bar	10	180	50%
Peanut Butter	1 bar	12	190	57%
Raisin	1 bar	9	170	48%

Food and Description	Amount	Fat Grams	Total Calories	% Fat Calories
(Nature Valley) Chocolate Chip	1 bar	4	110	33%
Peanut Butter	1 bar	6	120	45%
(Quaker) Chewy/Chocolate Chip	1 bar	5	130	35%
Honey & Oats	1 bar	4	125	29%
S'mores	1 bar	4	130	28%
Dipps/Caramel Nut	1 bar	6	150	36%
Chocolate Chip	1 bar	6	140	39%
Peanut Butter	1 bar	9	170	48%
(Ultra Slim Fast)				
Nutrition Dutch Chocolate	1 bar	4	140	26%
Snack/Chocolate Chip Crunch	1 bar	4	120	30%
GRAPEFRUIT				
Pink, White, & Red/canned				
in water	1/2 cup	0	44	0
in light syrup	1/2 cup	0	78	0
GRAPEFRUIT JUICE				
Boxed, Bottled, or Canned				
(Campbell's) Juice Bowl	6 oz	0	80	0
(Mott's) unsweetened	10 oz	0	124	0
(Sunkist) fresh squeezed	6 oz	0	56	0
Fresh	8 oz	0	96	0
From Frozen Concentrate	8 oz	0	102	0
GRAVY				
Canned & Jars/Au jus	1 can	.6	201	3%
Beef	1 can	6.8	156	39%
Brown	4 oz	6	94	57%
■ **GRAVY/DEHYDRATED MIXES: Prepared as Directed**				
Au jus	1 cup	.8	19	38%
Brown/(McCormick/Schilling)				
Au Jus	1/4 cup	< 1	20	23%
Brown, Lite	1/4 cup	1	10	90%
GREEN BEAN DISHES				
Bavarian Style (Birds Eye)	3.3 oz	6	110	49%
Cut Green Beans in Butter Sauce				
frozen (Green Giant)	1/2 cup	1	30	30%
GUM				
Bubble Yum/regular	1 piece	0	25	0
(Juicy Fruit)	1 stick	0	10	0

H

Food and Description	Amount	Fat Grams	Total Calories	% Fat Calories
HAM				
Canned-Black Label				
(Hormel)/1½ lb	4 oz	7	150	42%
Cured/regular	3 oz	11	163	61%
roasted	3 oz	13	194	60%
Cured-lean	3 oz	4	103	35%
Holiday Glaze Ham-3 lb	4 oz	4	130	28%
Minced	1 oz	5.86	75	70%
HAM AND CHEESE				
Loaf or Roll	1 oz	5.7	73	70%
Roll (Hormel)	4 oz	10	170	53%
Spread	1 Tbs	2.78	37	68%
HAM SALAD				
	1 Tbs	2	32	56%
	1 oz	4	61	59%
HAMBURGER HELPER				
(Betty Crocker) Box Mix, Prepared				
Beef Noodle	1 serv	15	330	41%
Cheddar'n Bacon	1 serv	19	380	45%
Cheeseburger Macaroni	1 serv	19	370	46%
Lasagna	1 serv	14	340	37%
Meat Loaf	1 serv	22	360	55%
Pizzabake	1 serv	14	320	39%
Sloppy Joe Bake	1 serv	15	340	40%
Spaghetti	1 serv	14	340	37%
Stroganoff	1 serv	20	390	46%
Tacobake	1 serv	15	320	42%
HICKORY NUT				
dried	1 oz	18	187	87%
HONEY				
	1 Tbs	0	64	0
	1/2 cup	0	512	0

Food and Description	Amount	Fat Grams	Total Calories	% Fat Calories
ICE CREAM				
(Breyers) Original/Chocolate	½ cup	8	160	45%
Mint Chocolate Chip	½ cup	10	170	53%
Strawberry	½ cup	6	130	42%
Vanilla	½ cup	8	150	48%
(Breyers) Light/Chocolate	½ cup	4	120	30%
Vanilla Raspberry Parfait	½ cup	3	130	21%
(Haagen-Dazs)/Chocolate	½ cup	17	270	57%
Coffee	½ cup	15	260	52%
Vanilla	½ cup	17	260	59%
(Sealtest)/Butter Pecan	½ cup	10	160	56%
Fudge Royale	½ cup	7	140	45%
Strawberry-Chocolate-Vanilla	½ cup	6	140	39%
(Weight Watchers) Grand Collection				
Strawberries'N Creme	½ cup	3	120	23%
Vanilla	½ cup	3	100	27%
ICE CREAM BAR & SANDWICH				
(Dove Bar)/Vanilla-Dark Choco.	1	22	340	58%
(Drumstick) Sundae Cone/Vanilla	1	19	332	52%
(Eskimo Pie)/Original Dark Choc.	1	12	140	71%
Fudge Bars-Sugar Free	1	1	60	15%
(Good Humor)/Chocolate Eclair	1	10	188	48%
Fudge Bar	1	< 1	127	4%
Vanilla-Chocolate Combo Cup	6 oz	9	201	40%
(Haagen-Dazs)/Vanilla-Dark	1 bar	27	360	68%
(Heath) Toffee Bars	1 bar	11	160	62%
(Klondike)/Chocolate	1 bar	20	287	63%
Vanilla	1 bar	20	294	61%
(Milky Way Bars) Chocolate	1 bar	11	190	52%
(Natural Nectar)/Cream Freezes				
Cocoa-Fudge'N Cream	1 bar	8	170	42%
(Oreo)/Sandwich	1	11	240	41%

Food and Description	Amount	Fat Grams	Total Calories	% Fat Calories
(Rondos)/Classic Vanilla	1 bar	4	60	60%
(Snickers)	1 bar	14	220	57%
(3 Musketeers)/Chocolate	1 bar	10	170	53%
ICE CREAM CONE				
Cones only/(Colosso) Cone	1	1.5	98	14%
(Disney) Waffle Cones	1 cone	< 1	59	8%
(Keebler)/Ice Cream Cups	1 cup	< 1	15	30%
Sugar Cones	1 cone	0	45	0
ICE CREAM TOPPING				
Butterscotch/(Smucker's)	2 Tbs	1	140	6%
Caramel/(Kraft)	1 Tbs	0	60	0
(Smucker's)	2 Tbs	1	140	6%
Cherry/(Smucker's)	1 Tbs	0	53	0
Chocolate Fudge/(Hershey)	2 Tbs	4	100	36%
Chocolate Syrup/(Hershey)	1 Tbs	0	36	0
(Nestle)	1.22 oz	1	100	9%
Hot Caramel/(Smucker's)	2 Tbs	4	150	24%
(Planter's) Nut Topping	1 oz	16	180	80%
Whipped Toppings/Frozen				
(Birds Eye) Cool Whip Lite	1 Tbs	<1	8	56%
(Kraft) Original	¼ cup	3	35	77%
(Reddi Whip) Lite	1 Tbs	< .5	6	45%
ICE MILK				
(Light N'Lively)/Chocolate Chip	½ cup	4	120	30%
Vanilla, Chocolate, Strawberry	½ cup	3	110	25%
(Weight Watchers)/One-Ders				
Chocolate Chip	4 oz	4	120	30%
Heavenly Hash	4 oz	3	130	21%
Strawberry	4 oz	3	110	25%
ICE MILK BAR				
(Crystal Light) Cool'N Creamy				
Bavarian Bar	1 bar	2	50	36%
Orange	1 bar	1	50	18%
(Kemps) Lite	1 bar	3	130	21%
(Sweet'N Low) Vanilla				
w/Chocolate Coating	1 bar	6	90	60%
(3 Musketeers)	1 bar	4	50	72%
(Weight Watchers)/Caramel Nut	1 bar	7	120	53%

J

Food and Description	Amount	Fat Grams	Total Calories	% Fat Calories
JAM/JELLY/PRESERVES				
(Kraft)/Jam &Jelly/all flavors	1 tsp	0	17	0
Preserves/reduced calorie				
Strawberry	1 tsp	0	8	0
(Nutradiet) sugar-free/Jam				
Strawberry	1 tsp	0	4	0
Jelly/Concord Grape	1 tsp	0	4	0
(R W Knudsen) All Fruit Spread				
Strawberry	2 tsp	0	35	0
(Smucker's)/Imitation Grape				
Jelly & Strawberry				
Jam (artificially sweetened)	1 tsp	0	2	0
Jam-all flavors	1 tsp	0	18	0
(Welch's)/Jams-all flavors	2 tsp	0	35	0
Jelly-all flavors	2 tsp	0	35	0

K

Food and Description	Amount	Fat Grams	Total Calories	% Fat Calories
KALE				
fresh-cooked	1/2 cup	0	21	0
KIDNEY BEAN				
Red/canned (B&M) baked	1 cup	7	290	22%
(Progresso)	8 oz	1	190	5%
KIWIFRUIT				
raw	1 large	<1	55	8%

L

Food and Description	Amount	Fat Grams	Total Calories	% Fat Calories
LAMB				
(NOTE: All portions are cooked, unless otherwise stated.				
Lean = all separable fat has been trimmed.				
Lean & fat = untrimmed and cooked as purchased.)				
Chop, arm/lean-braised	3 oz	14	270	47%
Chop, arm/lean & fat-braised	2.2 oz	15	220	61%
Chop, loin/lean-broiled	3 oz	8	182	40%
Chop, rib/lean-broiled	2 oz	7	130	49%
Chop, shoulder/lean-raw	7 oz	9	185	39%
Chop, shoulder/lean & fat-raw	7 oz	34	427	72%
Hocks	4 oz	16	236	61%
Leg, roast/lean-roasted	3 oz	7	162	39%
Leg, roast/lean & fat-roasted	3 oz	16	237	61%
Ribs/cooked-3 oz meat-raw	6 oz	8.9	178	45%
LAMB'S-QUARTERS				
fresh-cooked	1 cup	.6	29	19%
LARD	1 Tbs	12.8	115	100%
LASAGNA				
Frozen-w/meat sauce/(Banquet)	7 oz	10	270	33%
(Swanson's)	10.5 oz	16	400	36%
(Van de Kamp's) w/mushrooms	11 oz	25	430	52%
Vegetable Lasagna/(Weight Watchers)				
Italian Cheese Lasagna	11 oz	14	380	33%
w/ Meat Sauce	11 oz	13	330	36%
LEMON	1 medium	0	17	0
LEMONADE				
Bottled or canned/(Hi-C)	8.45 oz	0	109	0
(Tripicana) Single-Serve	8 oz	0	120	0
Frozen/(Birds Eye)	6 oz	0	70	0
(Minute Maid)	6 oz	0	77	0
Mix/(Country Time)/Pink				
Sugar-free	8 oz	0	4	0

Food and Description	Amount	Fat Grams	Total Calories	% Fat Calories
Sweetened	8 oz	0	80	0
LETTUCE				
Iceburg	1 head	1	70	13%
LICHEE (LYCHEE) NUTS				
dried/shelled	3 oz	.9	237	3%
LIMA BEAN				
Baby/raw	½ cup	1	330	3%
Canned/(Dennison's) w/ham	7.5 oz	7	250	25%
Frozen/(Green Giant)	1/2 cup	0	100	0
(Health Valley) thin	6 oz	.5	188	2%
Green/canned (Del Monte)	1/2 cup	0	70	0
LIMA BEAN DISHES				
In butter sauce				
frozen/(Green Giant)	1/2 cup	2	100	18%
LOBSTER				
Northern/boiled	3 oz	.5	83	5%
Spiny-raw	3 oz	1	95	10%
LUNCHEON MEAT				
(Butterball) Fresh Deli				
Oven Roasted Turkey Breast	1 slice	< 1	20	23%
Chicken Oven Roasted Breast				
(Weaver)	1 slice	.8	25	29%
Corned Beef				
Slender sliced (Eckrich)	1 oz	1	40	23%
(Healthy Choice)/Cold Cuts				
Baked Cooked Ham	2 oz	2	60	30%
Bologna	2 oz	2	60	30%
Oven Roasted Chicken	2 oz	1	60	15%
(Hillshire Farm) Bologna/large	1 oz	8	90	80%
Deli Select/Corned Beef	1 oz	< 1	31	15%
Pastrami	1 oz	< 1	30	15%
Flavorseal				
Beef Smoked Sausage	2 oz	16	180	80%
Lite Polska Kielbasa	2 oz	13	160	73%
Lite Smoked Sausage	2 oz	13	160	73%
Smoked Sausage-Italian	2 oz	18	200	81%
Kielbasa, Kalbassy Sausage				
Pork or Beef	1 oz	7.7	88	79%

Food and Description	Amount	Fat Grams	Total Calories	% Fat Calories
(Hormel) skinless	½ link	14	180	70%
Polska (Eckrich)-Lite	1 oz	6	70	77%
Skinless	1 oz	16	180	80%
Polska (Louis Rich)-turkey	1 oz	3	50	54%
Light & Lean (Hormel) Lunch Meats				
Bologna	2 slices	12	140	77%
Breast of Turkey	2 slices	2	60	30%
Canadian Style Bacon	2 slices	1	35	26%
Cooked Ham	2 slices	2	50	36%
Liver Sausage, Liverwurst/Pork	1 oz	8	93	77%
(Oscar Meyer) sliced	1 oz	9	95	85%
(Louis Rich) Cold Cuts				
Chopped Turkey Ham	1 slice	2	40	45%
(Oscar Meyer) Cold Cuts				
Beef-smoked-97% fat-free	1 slice	.5	15	30%
Bologna-Beef & Pork	1 oz	8	90	80%
Genoa Salami	1 slice	3	35	77%
Ham-boiled (96% fat-free)	1 slice	.5	25	18%
Head Cheese	1 slice	4	55	66%
Pepperoni/Pork, Beef	~ 9 oz	110	1248	79%
Pork/Slender sliced (Eckrich)	1 oz	2	45	40%
Salami/cooked-Beef	1 oz	5.9	74	72%
(Hormel)	2 slices	5	50	90%
(Hebrew National) beef-original				
deli style	1 oz	7	80	79%
Spam (Hormel)/luncheon	1¾ oz	14	150	84%
Turkey Breast Meat	~ 1.5 oz	.67	47	13%
Turkey Ham/(Butterball) Deli thin	1 oz	1	35	26%
Turkey Pastrami (Butterball)				
cold cuts	1 slice	1	30	30%
Turkey Roll-Light Meat	1 oz	2	42	43%
(Weight Watchers) Deli Meats				
Oven Roasted Beef	1 oz	1	30	90%
Oven Roasted Turkey t	1 oz	< 1	25	18%
Premium Baked Ham	1 oz	2	35	77%
Premium Bologna	1 oz	3	45	60%

M

Food and Description	Amount	Fat Grams	Total Calories	% Fat Calories
MACARONI AND CHEESE				
Canned	1 cup	9.6	228	38%
(Franco-American) frozen	7 oz.	9	220	37%
(Swanson's) frozen	10 oz.	21	400	47%
MACKEREL				
Atlantic/cooked-dry heat	3 oz	15	223	61%
Spanish/cooked-dry heat	3 oz	5	134	34%
MANDARIN ORANGE				
(Del Monte)	5.5 oz	< 1	100	5%
(Dole) Light Syrup	½ cup	< 1	76	6%
MANGO	1	.57	135	4%
diced/sliced	1 cup	.7	109	6%
MARGARINE/MARGARINE-LIKE SPREAD				
(Blue Bonnet)/Reduced Calorie	1 Tbs	6	50	100%
(Country Crock)/Original	1 Tbs	9	80	100%
(Fleischmann's)/Light Corn Oil Spread				
Soft or Stick	1 Tbs	8	80	100%
(I Can't Believe It's Not Butter)	1 Tbs	10	90	100%
Light Spread/Sticks	1 Tbs	7	60	100%
(Imperial)/Light	1 Tbs	6	60	100%
Soft	1 Tbs	11	100	100%
Whipped	1 Tbs	5.6	50	100%
(Kraft) Touch of Butter				
40% Fat-Tub	1 Tbs	6	50	100%
(Land O'Lakes)/Soft or Stick	1 tsp	4	35	100%
(Mazola)/Reduced Calorie				
Regular	1 Tbs	6	50	100%
(Parkay)/Liquid/Regular	1 Tbs	11	100	100%
(Promise)	1 Tbs	10	90	100%
Extra Light	1 Tbs	6	50	100%
(Shedd's)/Country Crock	1 Tbs	7	70	100%
(Touch of Butter) spread/stick	1 Tbs	10	90	100%

Food and Description	Amount	Fat Grams	Total Calories	% Fat Calories
(Weight Watchers) Spread	1 Tbs	4	45	100%
Regular	1 Tbs	6	50	100%
MARSHMALLOW				
(Campfire)	2	0	40	0
(Kraft) miniature	10	0	18	0
MATZO				
(Goodman's) Egg	1 piece	1	132	7%
(Manischewitz)				
Egg	10 crackers	2	108	17%
Whole Wheat w/bran	1 board	.6	110	5%
MATZO MEAL				
(Goodman's) Passover	1 cup	1	514	2%
MAYONNAISE				
(Hain)/Canola Light	1 Tbs	5	60	75%
Eggless	1 Tbs	12	110	98%
(Hellman's)	1 Tbs	11	100	100%
(Kraft) Cholesterol free	1 Tbs	10	90	100%
Light	1 Tbs	5	50	90%
Regular	1 Tbs	12	100	100%
(Miracle Whip) Free	1 Tbs	0	20	0
(Weight Watchers) Mayonnaise-Style Dressing				
Light	1 Tbs	5	50	90%
MEAT SUBSTITUTE				
Numette	2.5 oz	11	150	66%
Tender Cuts	2.2 oz	1	60	15%
MELBA TOAST				
(Devonsheer)/Garlic, Sesame, Onion				
Rye, Honey Bran	1 slice	0	12	0
White, Plain & Vegetable	1 slice	0	16	0
(Lance) Round-plain	2 slices	1	20	45%
Sesame	2 slices	1	25	36%
(Old London) Melba Toast				
Onion, White	3 slices	< 1	50	9%
Sesame	3 slices	< 2	50	36%
MEXICAN FOOD				
■ BEAN DIP				
Mexican (Hain)	4 Tbs	1	60	15%
Onion	4 Tbs	1	70	13%

Food and Description	Amount	Fat Grams	Total Calories	% Fat Calories
■ BURRITO				
Frozen (El Charrito)				
Bean & Cheese	5 oz	8	320	23%
Jalapeno Grande	6 oz	15	410	33%
(Old El Paso)/ Beef & Bean				
Medium	1	13	330	35%
Mild	1	11	320	31%
■ BURRITO FILLING/MIX				
(Del Monte)	½ cup	1	110	8%
■ CHILI & CHILI BEANS				
Beef Chili w/beans				
canned (Chef Boyardee)	7.5 oz	17	330	46%
Chili/canned				
Chicken/(Armour) Premium				
Lite w/Beans	7.5 oz	11	170	37%
Lentil/(Health Valley)	4 oz	5	110	41%
No Beans/(Hormel)	7⅜ oz	28	380	66%
(Libby's)	7.5 oz	30	390	69%
Extra Spicy	1 cup	21	330	57%
Frozen/(Banquet) Cookin' Bag				
Turkey	4 oz	2	80	23%
(Kraft) w/beef & beans	9.7 oz	22	380	52%
Microwave				
No Beans (Hormel)	10.5 oz	22	380	52%
Turkey (Healthy Choice)				
w/Beans	7.5 oz	5	200	23%
Vegetarian (Nile Spice)				
Chili'n Beans Mild	7 oz	1	160	6%
Mixes/(Hain)	¼ pkg	1	30	30%
Manwich Chili Fixins (Hunt's)				
Sauce Only	5.3 oz	1	110	8%
w/Regular Ground Beef	8 oz	14	290	43%
Chili Beans/canned				
Mexican Style (Van Camp's)	1 cup	2	210	9%
Chili con Carne/Canned (Heinz)	7¾ oz	21	350	54%
Canned w/ Beans (Chef Boyardee)				
Hot	7 oz	21	350	54%
Chili Sauce/(Del Monte)	¼ cup	1	70	13%

Food and Description	Amount	Fat Grams	Total Calories	% Fat Calories
■ **DINNER MIXES**				
(Old El Paso) Mexican Rice	½ cup	2	140	13%
■ **ENCHILADA SAUCE**				
Hot/(Old El Paso)	¼ cup	1	30	30%
Mix (Durkee)/Prepared	4 cups	2.4	229	9%
■ **ENCHILADAS**				
Beef/Box mix (International Lites)				
Enchilada Acapulco-prepared	10 oz	8	250	29%
Beef/frozen (Hormel)	1	5	140	32%
(Old El Paso)	2	10	170	53%
Cheese/frozen				
(3) (El Charrito)	11 oz	20	470	38%
Chicken/frozen				
Chicken Enchilada	½ pkg	11	260	38%
■ **FAJITAS**				
Frozen (Weight Watchers)/Beef	6.75 oz	7	250	25%
Chicken	6.75 oz	5	270	21%
■ **FROZEN ENTREE/DINNER**				
(Banquet)				
Chili Gravy & Beef Enchiladas	7 oz	13	270	43%
Family Entrees/Chili Sauce				
w/Beef & Beef Enchilada	7 oz	13	270	43%
Meals & Platters				
Chimichanga	9.5 oz	9	480	17%
Mexican Style	11 oz	17	410	37%
(El Charrito)				
Beef Enchilada Dinner	13.75 oz	31	620	45%
Cheese Enchilada Dinner	13.25 oz	24	570	38%
(Van de Kamp's)/Mexican-Style	½ pkg	10	220	41%
■ **NACHO SAUCE**				
(Kaukauna) Cheese	1 oz	6	80	68%
■ **NACHOS**				
Muy Fresco/Frozen-microwave	3.5 oz	9	140	51%
■ **REFRIED BEANS**				
Canned (Del Monte)/Plain	½ cup	2	130	14%
(Hain)/Vegetarian	4 oz	1	70	13%
■ **TACO SEASONING MIX**				
(Old El Paso) Mix Only	1/12 pkg	< 1	8	56%
(Ortega)/Mix Only	1 oz	1	90	10%

Food and Description	Amount	Fat Grams	Total Calories	% Fat Calories
Prepared as Directed	1 oz	4	60	60%
■ TACO SHELLS				
(Old El Paso)	1 shell	3	55	49%
(Ortega)	1 shell	2	50	36%
■ TACOS				
Beef/Hamburger Helper				
(Betty Crocker) Tacobake				
Box Mix/Dry	⅙ pkg	4	170	21%
Box Mix/Prepared	⅙ recipe	15	320	42%
Taco Starter/(Del Monte)	8 oz	1	140	6%
■ TORTILLA				
Corn/(El Charrito)	2	1	95	10%
(Old El Paso)	1	1	60	15%
■ TOSTACO SHELLS				
Corn (Old El Paso)	1 shell	5	100	45%
MILK				
Buttermilk/Cultured	1 cup	2	99	18%
Carob-Chocolate Milk 1%	1 cup	3	160	17%
Chocolate/Low-Fat 2%/(Hershey)	1 cup	5	180	25%
(Nestle)	1 cup	9	210	39%
Condensed/canned-sweetened	¼ cup	6.6	244	24%
(Carnation)	1 oz	3	123	22%
Fresh/Low-fat 2%	1 cup	5	121	37%
Low-fat 1%	1 cup	2.6	105	22%
Skim	1 cup	.6	100	6%
Whole/(Real) Real Fresh milk w/vitamins				
A & D-ready to chill box	1 cup	8	150	48%
MILK MIXES				
Chocolate/(Choco Milk) dry mix	1 oz	1	110	8%
+ 8 oz whole milk	8 oz	10	264	34%
Chocolate syrup	2 Tbs	.5	82	6%
+ whole milk	8 oz	8.5	232	33%
Cocoa/(Carnation)				
Chocolate Fudge-dry	1 oz	1	110	8%
Diet Hot Cocoa Mix	1 env	< 1	25	18%
(Nestle Quik)/Chocolate				
+ 8 oz whole milk	8 oz	9	240	34%
+ 8 oz 2% milk	8 oz	6	210	26%

Food and Description	Amount	Fat Grams	Total Calories	% Fat Calories
_+ 8 oz skim milk	8 oz	1.6	180	8%
(Swiss Miss) instant				
Chocolate Mint	1 pkt	3	150	18%
Mini Marshmallow	1 pkt	1	110	8%
Sugar Free	1 pkt	1	60	15%
Malted/(Ovaltine) Classic-Traditional Chocolate Malt				
_w/2% milk	8 oz	5	210	21%
Strawberry (Nestle Quik)				
+ 8 oz whole milk	8 oz	8	230	31%
+ 8 oz 2% milk	8 oz	5	200	23%
MUFFINS				
(Betty Crocker)/Mix only				
Apple Cinnamon	1	3	100	27%
Oat Bran	1	7	170	37%
(Duncan Hines) mix				
Bakery Style Cinnamon Swirl	1	7	200	32%
(Entenmann's) Blueberry	1	8	200	36%
(Flako) Corn mix	1	4	120	30%
(Health Valley) Fat Free fruit	1	< 1	65	7%
Oat Bran Almond-Date	1	6	170	32%
(Hostess) Breakfast Bake Shop				
Oat Bran Banana Nut	1	5	140	32%
(Krusteaz) mix/Cornbread	1	7	220	29%
(Thomas)/Plain & Sourdough	1	1	120	8%
Raisin	1	1.5	153	4%
(Sara Lee) Frozen/Corn	1	13	250	47%
MUSHROOM				
Canned/(B&B)	2 oz	1	25	36%
(Libby's)	1 oz	0	70	0
Fresh-Boiled	½ cup	0	21	0
Frozen (Freshlike)	1	0	9	0
MUSHROOM DISHES				
Mushroom Stroganoff (Light Balance)				
Microwaveable	8.25 oz	5	180	25%
Mushrooms breaded-frozen				
(Ore Ida)	2⅔ oz	8	140	51%
Mushrooms w/butter sauce				
canned	2 oz	1	30	30%

Food and Description	Amount	Fat Grams	Total Calories	% Fat Calories
MUSTARD				
Brown/(Heinz)	1 tsp	< 1	8	56%
(Nabisco)	1 tsp	0	4	0
Prepared/(French's)				
Bold & Spicy	1 tsp	< 1	6	75%
Dijon	1 tsp	< 1	8	56%
Grey Poupon/(Nabisco)	1 tsp	1	18	50%
(Gulden's)/Spicy Brown	1 Tbs	< 1	9	50%
(Heinz)/Mild	1 tsp	0	5	0
Horseradish	1 Tbs	1	14	64%
(Kraft)/Pure Prepared	1 Tbs	1	11	82%

N

Food and Description	Amount	Fat Grams	Total Calories	% Fat Calories
NUTRITIONAL SUPPLEMENTS				
(Carnation) Slender-All Flavors	10 oz	4	220	16%
(Dynatrim) Mix-Dry				
Dutch Chocolate	1 serv.	1	100	9%
Vanilla Royale	1 serv.	1	100	9%
(Ultra Slim Fast) Canned-Original/Liquid				
Chocolate Royale	11 oz	3	230	12%
French Vanilla	11 oz	3	210	13%
Powder/Chocolate Malt	1 scoop	< 1	100	5%
w/8 oz skim milk	8 oz	1	190	5%
Strawberry Jubilee	1 scoop	1	110	8%
w/8 oz skim milk	8 oz	2	240	8%
(Ultra Slim Fast) Water-Mixable Shake Mix				
Dutch Chocolate	1 envl	< 1	220	2%
French Vanilla	1 envl	< 1	220	2%
(Weight Watchers)/Shake Mix				
Chocolate Fudge	1 pkt	1	70	13%

Food and Description	Amount	Fat Grams	Total Calories	% Fat Calories
Orange Sherbet	1 pkt	0	70	0
NUTS, MIXED				
Mixed Nuts/(Eagle)	1 oz	16	180	80%
(Planters)/Dry Roasted	1 oz	14	160	79%
Unsalted	1 oz	15	170	79%
Oil Roasted	1 oz	16	180	80%
Select Mix/Cashews w/Almonds & Peanuts	1 oz	14	170	74%
Mixed Nuts w/Peanuts				
Dry Roasted	1 oz	14.6	169	78%
Oil Roasted	1 oz	16	175	82%
Mixed Nuts w/o Peanuts				
Oil Roasted	1 oz	15.95	175	82%

O

Food and Description	Amount	Fat Grams	Total Calories	% Fat Calories
OATS				
(Arrowhead Mills)/Flakes	2 oz	4	220	16%
Whole Grain	1 oz	2	110	16%
OCEAN PERCH, ATLANTIC				
Breaded & fried	3 oz	11	185	54%
Cooked-dry heat	3 oz	1.8	103	16%
Mixed/Frozen-raw (Gorton's)	5 oz	1	110	8%
OCTOPUS/ raw	3 oz	.88	70	11%
OILS				
ALL VEGETABLE OILS	1 Tbs	14	120	100%

[NOTE: You need to watch even your use of "healthier"(less saturated) oils, in order to keep your total fat intake within acceptable boundaries. Because it is so important for you to select the least saturated oil to fit your needs, I have listed the most commonly used oils and fats below, showing the % of saturated fat, polyunsaturated fat, and monounsaturated fat in each one. Those that contain less satu-

Food and Description	Amount	Fat Grams	Total Calories	% Fat Calories

rated fat are listed first for both oils and fats. (Data is based on information from USDA Nutritive Value of American Foods in Common Units, 1988.)]

REMEMBER—NO VEGETABLE OIL CONTAINS CHOLESTEROL!

■ OILS & FATS

VEGETABLE OIL/FAT	% SATURATED	% UNSATURATED % POLY	% MONO
CANOLA	7	35	58
SAFFLOWER	9	78	13
SUNFLOWER	11	69	20
CORN	13	62	25
OLIVE	14	12	74
SOYBEAN	15	43	42
MARGARINE/(Liquid/Tub)	17	37	46
(Stick)	20	33	47
PEANUT	18	33	49
WHEAT GERM	20	50	31
SHORTENING (VEGETABLE)	27	26	47
COCOA BUTTER	62	3	35
BUTTER/(Stick)	66	4	30
(Whipped)	69	3	28
COCONUT	92	2	6

ANIMAL FAT	% SATURATED	% UNSATURATED
CHICKEN	30	70
TURKEY	30	70
DUCK	34	66
SALT PORK	36	64
LARD	41	59
BEEF TALLOW	52	48

OLIVE
Pickled/canned or bottled

Food and Description	Amount	Fat Grams	Total Calories	% Fat Calories
Green	10 Small	3.6	33	98%

Food and Description	Amount	Fat Grams	Total Calories	% Fat Calories
Pitted Ripe/(S&W)-Jumbo	3.5 oz	18	163	99%
ONION DISHES				
Onion Ringers/frozen (Ore Ida)	2 oz	7	140	45%
Onion Rings/Frozen, Breaded				
(Mrs. Paul's) Crispy	2.5 oz	12	190	57%
Small Onions w/cream sauce/frozen				
(Birds Eye)	3 oz	6	110	49%
ORIENTAL FOOD				
Frozen (Van de Kamp's)	11 oz	10	310	29%
■ **(BETTY CROCKER) BOX MIX**				
Skillet Chicken Helper, Stir-Fried	⅕ box	11	330	30%
■ **CHOW MEIN**				
Beef, canned	¾ cup	1	70	13%
Chicken, canned	¾ cup	3	80	34%
■ **(CHUN KING)**				
Egg Rolls & Side Dishes/Frozen				
Chicken Egg Rolls	3.5 oz	7	210	30%
Fried Rice w/Chicken	8 oz	4	254	14%
Fried Rice w/Pork	8 oz	5	263	17%
Meat & Shrimp Egg Rolls	3.5 oz	8	214	34%
Entrees/Frozen				
Beef Pepper Oriental	13 oz	3	310	9%
Chicken Chow Mein	13 oz	6	370	10%
Imperial Chicken	13 oz	1	300	3%
Stir-Fry Entrees/Canned-Prepared				
Chow Mein w/chicken	6 oz	11	220	45%
Egg Foo Young	5 oz	8	140	51%
Pepper Steak	6 oz	17	250	61%
■ **EGG ROLL**				
frozen (Chun King)				
Meat & Shrimp	3.6 oz	8	220	33%
Shrimp	3.6 oz	6	200	27%
■ **(HUNT'S) MINUTE GOURMET**				
Oriental Beef/box mix-prep	6.4 oz	14	290	43%
Sweet & Sour Chicken/box	7.8 oz	4	300	12%
■ **(LA CHOY) Canned Chow Meins**				
Beef	¾ cup	1	60	15%
Chicken	¾ cup	2	70	26%

Food and Description	Amount	Fat Grams	Total Calories	% Fat Calories
Shrimp	¾ cup	1	45	20%
Entrees/Beef Pepper Oriental	¾ cup	2	90	20%
Sweet & Sour Oriental				
w/chicken	¾ cup	2	240	8%
w/pork	¾ cup	4	250	14%
■ (LEAN CUISINE)				
Chicken Chow Mein	9 oz	5	240	19%
Oriental Beef	8.5 oz	7	250	25%
■ (LEAN POCKETS)				
Chicken Oriental/frozen	1	6	250	22%
■ SZECHWAN CHICKEN				
(International Lites)	10 oz	5	270	17%
■ TERIYAKI CHICKEN				
canned-prepared	¾ cup	2	85	21%
■ (TYSON) Gourmet Selection Entrees				
Chicken Oriental	10.25 oz	7	270	23%
Sweet & Sour Chicken	11 oz	16	440	33%
Teriyaki Chicken	11 oz	2	130	14%
Teriyaki Chicken Wings	11 oz	14	220	57%
Stir Fry/Frozen				
Chicken Stir Fry	4 oz	6	130	42%
Resolutions Beef Stir Fry	5.6 oz	4	180	20%

P

Food and Description	Amount	Fat Grams	Total Calories	% Fat Calories
PANCAKE				
■ FROZEN				
(Aunt Jemima)/Blueberry	3	4	200	18%
Buttermilk	3	2	180	10%
(Downyflake)/Blueberry	3	9	290	28%
Regular	3	9	280	29%
(Krusteaz)/Buttermilk	3	5	290	16%

Food and Description	Amount	Fat Grams	Total Calories	% Fat Calories
■ FROZEN MICROWAVEABLE				
(Aunt Jemima)/Blueberry	3	4	220	16%
Buttermilk	3	3	210	13%
Buttermilk Lite	3	3	140	19%
(Swanson-Great Starts)				
Pancakes & Sausages	6 oz	22	460	43%
Silver Dollar cakes & Sausage	3¾ oz	14	310	41%
Whole Wheat cakes w/ Links	5.5 oz	16	350	41%
PANCAKE BATTER				
Frozen/(Aunt Jemima)				
Blueberry	3.6 oz	4	204	18%
Buttermilk	3.6 oz	2	180	10%
PANCAKE/WAFFLE MIX				
(Arrowhead Mills)/Griddle Lite	½ cup	3	260	10%
Multi-grain	½ cup	2	350	5%
(Aunt Jemima)/Buckwheat	3	1.6	143	10%
Buttermilk Pancake & Waffle	3	< 1	122	5%
Complete Buttermilk	3	3	230	12%
Lite	3	2	130	14%
Original Pancake & Waffle	3	< 1	116	6%
No cholesterol version	3	4	170	21%
(Bisquick)/Shake'N Pour				
Blueberry	3	3	270	10%
Original	3	4	250	14%
(Hungry Jack)/Buttermilk				
w/Egg	3	9	210	39%
w/Egg Whites	3	7	200	32%
Buttermilk Complete	3	3	180	15%
PASTA				
(Contadina) Fresh Chilled w/o Sauce				
Angel's Hair	3 oz	3	260	10%
Fettucine (Spinach)	3 oz	4	260	14%
Ravioli/w/Beef	3 oz	3	270	10%
w/Cheese	3 oz	11	270	37%
w/Meat	3 oz	6	260	21%
Tortellini/w/Cheese (Egg)	3 oz	6	260	21%
(Creamette) Dry				
Enriched Elbow Macaroni	2 oz	1	210	4%

Food and Description	Amount	Fat Grams	Total Calories	% Fat Calories
Enriched Spaghetti	2 oz	1	210	4%
Enriched Wide Egg Noodles	2 oz	3	220	12%
(Mueller's) Dry				
Egg Noodles	2 oz	3	220	12%
Tri-Color Twists	2 oz	1	210	4%
Noodles/Chow Mein				
Dry (La Choy)	½ cup	8	150	48%
Egg/Cooked	1 cup	2	200	9%
Oriental Noodles/Chinese				
(Chun King)/Canned	1 oz	7	140	45%
(Ronzoni) Dry				
Egg Noodles	2 oz	2	210	9%
Spinach	2 oz	3	220	12%
Macaroni	2 oz	< 1	210	2%
Tri-color Rotini	2 oz	1	210	4%
(San Giorgio) Dry				
Cut Ziti	1 oz	<1	110	4%
Light & Fluffy/Egg Noodles				
Spinach	1 oz	2	110	16%
Spaghetti	1 oz	<1	110	4%
(Weight Watchers) Dry				
Elbow Style	2 oz	1	160	6%
(Westbrae Natural) Whole Wheat-Dry				
Lasagna	2 oz	2	210	9%
Spaghettii	2 oz	2	210	9%
PASTA ENTREE/DINNER				
(Betty Crocker) Mix				
Presto Pasta/Creamy Alfredo	¼ pkg	18	370	44%
Suddenly Salad/Caesar Dry	⅙ pkg	1	110	8%
Prepared	½ cup	8	170	42%
Creamy Macaroni/Dry	⅙ pkg	< 1	100	5%
Prepared	½ cup	10	200	45%
Prepared-lower fat recipe	½ cup	4	140	26%
Italian Pasta/Dry	⅙ pkg	1	110	8%
Prepared	½ cup	6	160	34%
Pasta Primavera/Dry	⅙ pkg	< 1	90	5%
Prepared	½ cup	10	190	47%
Prepared-lower fat recipe	½ cup	5	150	30%

Food and Description	Amount	Fat Grams	Total Calories	% Fat Calories
(Chef Boy Ar Dee)				
Canned/ABC's & 1,2,3's				
w/Mini Meatballs	7.5 oz	9	240	34%
in Sauce	7.5 oz	1	160	6%
Beefaroni	7.5 oz	8	220	33%
Dinosaurs w/Meatballs	8.6 oz	11	280	35%
Ravioli Products/Cheese Ravioli				
in Beef & Tomato Sauce	7.5 oz	3	200	14%
Spaghetti & Meatballs				
w/tomato sauce-15 oz	7.5 oz	9	230	35%
(Franco-American)/Canned				
Beef Ravioli's in Meat Sauce	7.5 oz	8	250	29%
Macaroni & Cheese	7 3/8 oz	5	170	27%
Spaghettio's in Tomato				
& Cheese Sauce	7.5 oz	2	170	7%
Spaghettio's w/Meatballs				
in Tomato Sauce	7⅜ oz	8	210	66%
(Green Giant) Frozen				
Entrees/Lasagna	12 oz	20	490	37%
Macaroni & Cheese	9 oz	10	290	31%
Pasta Accents				
Cheddar Cheese Seasoning	½ cup	3	90	30%
Garlic Seasoning	½ cup	4	100	36%
Primavera	½ cup	4	110	33%
(Healthy Choice)/Canned				
Lasagna w/Meat Sauce	7.5 oz	5	220	20%
Spaghetti w/Meat Sauce	7.5 oz	3	150	18%
(Kraft) Mix/Dinners-Prepared				
Macaroni & Cheese	¾ cup	13	290	40%
Deluxe	¾ cup	8	260	28%
Spaghetti Dinner				
American Style	1 cup	7	300	21%
w/Meat Sauce	1 cup	14	360	35%
Pasta & Cheese-prepared				
Cheddar Broccoli	½ cup	8	180	40%
Chicken w/Herbs	½ cup	7	170	37%
Fettuccine Alfredo	½ cup	9	180	45%
3-Cheese & Vegetable	½ cup	8	180	40%

Food and Description	Amount	Fat Grams	Total Calories	% Fat Calories
PASTRY, TOASTER				
(Kellogg's) Pop Tarts				
Frosted blueberry	1	6	210	26%
Frosted chocolate fudge	1	5	200	23%
Frosted Cinnamon	1	7	210	30%
Frosted strawberry	1	5	200	23%
(Nabisco) Toastettes Pastry				
Apple	1	5	190	24%
Frosted/Fudge	1	5	200	23%
Strawberry	1	5	190	24%
(Pepperidge Farm) Toaster Tarts				
Apple Cinnamon	1	7	170	37%
Cheese	1	10	190	47%
Strawberry	1	7	190	33%
(Pillsbury) Toaster Muffins				
Apple Spice	1	5	130	35%
Raisin bran	1	5	120	38%
Toaster Strudel Breakfast Pastry				
Apple spice, Blueberry, Cinnamon,				
Raspberry, Strawberry	1	8	190	38%
Cherry	1	9	190	43%
PEA DISHES				
Early Peas in Butter Sauce				
frozen micro (Green Giant)	4.5 oz	2	80	23%
Green peas in cream sauce				
frozen (Birds Eye)	2.6 oz	6	120	45%
Green peas, potatoes in cream sauce				
frozen (Bird's Eye)	2.6 oz	6	130	42%
Peas in Butter Sauce				
frozen Micro Quick (Freshlike)	5 oz	2	110	16%
Sweet Peas in Butter Sauce				
frozen (Green Giant)	½ cup	2	80	23%
PEANUT				
■ **ALL TYPES**				
Boiled	½ cup	7	102	62%
Dry Roasted	1 oz	13.9	164	76%
Lite	1 oz	9	135	60%
Honey Roasted	1 oz	13	170	69%

Food and Description	Amount	Fat Grams	Total Calories	% Fat Calories
PEANUT BUTTER				
■ CHUNKY				
(Peter Pan)	2 Tbs	16	180	80%
Creamy	2⅔ Tbs	16	190	76%
Crunchy	2⅔ Tbs	16	190	76%
(Skippy) Super Chunk	2 Tbs	17	190	81%
(Smucker's) Natural	2 Tbs	16	200	72%
■ CREAMY/SMOOTH				
(Arrowhead Mills)	2 Tbs	16	190	76%
(Jiff)	2 Tbs	16	190	76%
(Peter Pan)	2 Tbs	16	180	80%
(Skippy)	2 Tbs	17	190	81%
■ CRUNCHY				
(Arrowhead Mills)	2 Tbs	16	190	76%
(Jif) 2 Tbs	17	190	81%	
(Peter Pan)	2 Tbs	16	180	80%
(Skippy)/Roasted Honey Nut	2 Tbs	17	190	81%
■ MIXED				
(Smucker's)				
w/ fudge/Goober Fudge	2 Tbs	13	240	49%
w/ honey/Goober Honey	2 Tbs	10	180	50%
w/ jelly/Goober Grape	2 Tbs	10	180	50%
■ NO-SALT NATURAL				
(Smuckers)	2 Tbs	17	200	77%
PEANUT BUTTER FLAVORED BAKING CHIPS				
(Reese's)	¼ cup	13	230	51%
PEAR				
Canned/in Water	1 cup	< 1	71	6%
in Juice	1 cup	< 1	123	4%
in Heavy Syrup	1 cup	< 1	188	2%
(S&W) Bartlett Halves in				
Heavy Syrup	1/2 cup	0	100	0
Natural-Sliced	1/2 cup	0	80	0
PECAN				
(Azar) Chips	1 oz	21	210	90%
Dry Roasted	1 oz	18	187	87%
(Eagle) Honey Roasted	1 oz	19	200	86%
(Planters) Halves	1 oz	20	190	95%

Food and Description	Amount	Fat Grams	Total Calories	% Fat Calories
PEPPER DISHES				
Standard Home Recipe (USDA)				
Stuffed Green Pepper				
w/ beef & bread crumbs	1 med	10.5	325	29%
PICKLE				
Bread & butter pickles	3 slices	0	16	0
(Del Monte) Dill Halves	1 oz	0	4	0
(Vlasic) Bread &Butter Chunks	1 oz	0	25	0
PIE & COBBLER				
Apple (Mrs. Smith's)				
Old Fashioned	⅛ pie	27	530	46%
Ready to Bake	⅛ pie	17	390	39%
(Weight Watchers)-frozen	3.5 oz	4	165	22%
Boston Cream-frozen				
(Mrs. Smith's) Thaw'N Serve	⅛ pie	4	240	15%
(Weight Watchers)	3 oz	4	190	19%
Cherry/(Banquet)-frozen	3.33 oz	11	250	40%
(Mrs. Smith's)-frozen				
Old Fashioned	⅛ pie	19	460	37%
Chocolate/frozen (Banquet)	2.33 oz	10	185	49%
Chocolate Cream-frozen				
(Mrs. Smith's) Thaw'N Serve	⅛ pie	13	270	43%
Coconut Custard/frozen				
(Mrs. Smith's) Ready Bake	⅛ pie	15	330	41%
Lemon Meringue/frozen				
(Mrs. Smith's) Thaw'N Serve	⅛ pie	6	290	19%
Pumpkin/frozen (Banquet)	3.33 oz	8	200	36%
Snack-packaged				
(Hostess) Apple	1	20	430	42%
Cherry	1	20	460	39%
(Hostess) Pudding Pies				
Chocolate	1	19	490	35%
Vanilla	1	17	470	33%
(Little Debbie) Marshmallow pies				
Banana	9 oz	12	360	30%
Chocolate	3 oz	13	370	32%
(Tastykake) Apple	1 pkg	12	300	36%
Cherry	1 pkg	10	300	30%

Food and Description	Amount	Fat Grams	Total Calories	% Fat Calories
PIE CRUST				
(Flako) (9" dia)	1/6 crust	15	250	54%
(Keebler) Ready Crust				
Butter flavored	1/8 crust	5	110	41%
Graham Cracker	1/8 crust	6	120	45%
(Krusteaz) baked	~1 oz	6	100	54%
(Pillsbury) Mix	1/8 crust	13	200	59%
Refrigerated-all ready	1/8 crust	15	240	56%
PIE FILLING				
■ PIE FILLING-CREAM-CANNED				
(Comstock) Banana	3.5 oz	2	110	16%
Chocolate	3.5 oz	3	130	21%
Coconut	3.5 oz	3	120	23%
Lemon	3.5 oz	1	140	13%
■ PIE FILLING-FRUIT				
Canned/(Comstock)				
(Libby's)/Baked	1/6 pie	17	330	46%
(Libby's)/Pumpkin	1 cup	0	210	0
■ PIE FILLING-INSTANT				
Mixes prepared w/whole milk (Jell-O)				
Chocolate	1/2 cup	4	130	28%
Coconut cream	1/2 cup	6	180	30%
Lemon	1/2 cup	4	140	26%
■ PIE FILLING-INSTANT SUGAR-FREE				
Mixes prepared w/2% low-fat milk (Jell-O)				
Chocolate	1/2 cup	3	100	27%
Vanilla	1/2 cup	2	90	20%
■ PIE FILLING-MIX				
Prepared w/whole milk				
(Jell-O)/Banana cream (8" pie)				
Chocolate	1/2 cup	5	180	25%
Vanilla	1/2 cup	4	160	23%
■ PIE FILLING-MIX-SUGAR-FREE				
Prepared w/2% milk (Jell-O)				
Chocolate	1/2 cup	3	90	30%
Vanilla	1/2 cup	2	80	30%
PISTACHIO NUT				
(Planters)/dry roasted	1 oz	15	170	79%

Food and Description	Amount	Fat Grams	Total Calories	% Fat Calories
red	1 oz	15	170	79%
PIZZA & PIZZA SNACK				
■ (CELENTANO)				
9-slice pizza	2.7 oz	4	150	24%
ThickCrust Pizza	4.3	11	290	34%
(CELESTE)				
Original/Cheese	¼ pizza	17	315	49%
Deluxe	¼ pizza	22	380	52%
Pepperoni	¼ pizza	29	370	71%
Sausage	¼ pizza	22	375	53%
■ (CHEF BOY-AR-DEE)				
Box Mix/Cheese Pizza	3.84 oz	6	230	24%
Pepperoni Pizza	3.38 oz	6	230	24%
Sausage Pizza	4.22 oz	10	270	33%
■ (ELIO'S) HEALTHY SLICE				
Mixed Vegetable	3.1 oz	2	150	12%
Cheese	5.6 oz	3	300	9%
Pepperoni	6.25 oz	8	320	23%
■ (HEALTHY CHOICE) FRENCH BREAD PIZZA				
Cheese	5.6 oz	3	300	9%
Deluxe	6.25 oz	8	330	22%
Pepperoni	6.25 oz	8	320	23%
■ (JENO'S)				
Crisp 'n Tasty Pizza				
Cheese(7.4 oz)	½ pizza	10	240	38%
Combination(7.8 oz)	½ pizza	15	280	48%
Pizza Rolls/Cheese	3 oz	5	200	23%
Pepperoni	3 oz	9	220	37%
■ (LEAN CUISINE)				
French Bread Pizza				
Cheese	5⅛ oz	9	300	27%
Deluxe	6⅛ oz	8	320	23%
Pepperoni	5¼ oz	11	330	30%
■ (LEAN POCKETS)				
Pizza Deluxe				
w/pepperoni & sausage	1 pocket	13	280	42%
■ SNACK TRAY PIZZA				
Cheese (12)	4 pizzas	7	130	49%
Pepperoni (12)	4 pizzas	8	140	51%

Food and Description	Amount	Fat Grams	Total Calories	% Fat Calories
■ (STOUFFER'S)				
French Bread Pizza				
Cheese (10 3/8 oz)	1/2 pizza	14	350	36%
Deluxe (12⅜ oz)	½ pizza	19	420	41%
Sausage & Pepperoni (12.5 oz)'	1/2 pizza	23	460	45%
Pepperoni (11¼ oz)	½ pizza	19	400	43%
Vegetable Deluxe (12.75 oz)	1/2 pizza	20	420	43%
■ (TOMBSTONE)				
Double Top 12"				
Pepperoni w/Double Cheese	4.8 oz	20	360	50%
Italian Style Thin Crust				
Cheese & Pepperoni	3.04 oz	14	230	55%
Mexican Style Thin Crust				
Ranchero Deluxe	3.4 oz	13	230	51%
Microwave 7"/Cheese	7.7 oz	24	500	43%
Sausage & Pepperoni	8 oz	32	570	51%
Original 9"/Cheese	5.6 oz	17	380	40%
■ (TONY'S)				
French Bread/Cheese	5.5 oz	8	360	20%
Pepperoni	5.9 oz	15	430	31%
Supreme	6.3 oz	13	420	28%
Microwave/Sausage & Pepperoni	3.5 oz	17	300	51%
■ (WEIGHT WATCHERS)				
French Bread Pizza/Deluxe	5.94 oz	7	260	24%
Pizza/Cheese	6.03 oz	7	300	21%
Sausage	6.43 oz	10	340	26%
POPCORN				
(Eagle) Ready-to-Eat				
Cheese & White Cheddar	½ oz	6	80	68%
(Jiffy Pop) Popped/Bag				
Butter/Light	3 cups	3	80	34%
Regular	3 cups	5	100	45%
Microwave/Butter	4 cups	7	140	45%
(Jolly Time) Microwave/Butter	3 cups	5	90	50%
Light	3 cups	2	60	30%
Cheddar Cheese	3 cups	11	180	55%
Regular/White-no butter	4 cups	.6	77	7%
(Newman's Own)Butter	3 cups	8	150	48%

Food and Description	Amount	Fat Grams	Total Calories	% Fat Calories
(Orville Redenbacher's)				
Microwave/Butter/Popped	3 cups	6	100	54%
Caramel/Popped	3 cups	14	240	53%
Light/Butter/Popped	3 cups	3	70	39%
Popcorn Snack Cakes				
(Smartfood)/Cheddar Cheese	½ oz	5	80	56%
Light Butter	½ oz	3	70	39%
(Wise)				
Tender Eating Baby Popcorn	.5 oz	6	70	77%
w/Real White Cheddar	.5 oz	5	70	64%

PORK (*See also* BACON, HAM, LUNCHEON MEAT, SAUSAGE)

(NOTE: The information listed below on "Today's Leaner Pork" was provided by the National Pork, Livestock, and Meat Board. Following this is information on "Miscellaneous Cuts," which was provided by the United States Department of Agriculture. Please note that the data listed under "Today's Leaner Pork" apply to meat that has been roasted and trimmed of all separable fat.)

■ **TODAY'S LEANER PORK**

Food and Description	Amount	Fat Grams	Total Calories	% Fat Calories
Blade Steaks	3 oz	10.7	193	50%
Center Loin Chop	3 oz	6.9	165	38%
Center Rib Chop	3 oz	8.5	179	43%
Loin Chops	3 oz	6.9	172	36%
Loin Chops (Boneless)	3 oz	6.6	173	34%
Loin Roast (Boneless)	3 oz	6	165	33%
Rib Roast (Boneless)	3 oz	8.6	182	43%
Ribs (Country Style)	3 oz	12.6	210	54%
Sirloin Chops (Boneless)	3 oz	5.7	164	31%
Sirloin Roast	3 oz	8.7	184	43%
Tenderloin	3 oz	4	139	26%

POTATO

White/frozen

Food and Description	Amount	Fat Grams	Total Calories	% Fat Calories
cottage cut/cooked in oven	10 pieces	4	109	33%
fried in vegetable oil	10 pieces	8	158	46%

POTATO CHIPS

Food and Description	Amount	Fat Grams	Total Calories	% Fat Calories
(Eagle)/Barbeque Flavored	1 oz	8	150	48%
Sour Cream & Onion	1 oz	10	150	60%
(Lay's)/Bar B Q	1 oz	9	150	54%
Original	1 oz	10	150	60%
Sour Cream & Onion	1 oz	10	160	56%

Food and Description	Amount	Fat Grams	Total Calories	% Fat Calories
(New York Deli)	1 oz	11	160	62%
(Pringle's)/BBQ	1 oz	11	160	62%
(Ruffles)/Original	1 oz	10	150	60%
Sour Cream & Onions	1 oz	10	160	56%
(Wise) Natural	1 oz	11	160	62%
Ridges-Barbecue	1 oz	10	150	60%
POTATO DISHES				
Au Gratin/box mix	1 cup	10	230	39%
frozen (Banquet)	½ cup	2	98	18%
Baked-Frozen				
(Healthy Choice)/ Broccoli & Cheese Sauce				
w/Baked Potato Wedges	9.5 oz	5	240	23%
(Weight Watchers)				
Broccoli & Cheese	10.5 oz	6	270	20%
Chicken Divan	11.25 oz	7	280	23%
(Betty Crocker) box mixes				
Microwave-prepared				
Au Gratin	1 serving	5	140	24%
Scalloped	1 serving	5	140	32%
Sour Cream & Chive	1 serving	5	140	39%
Escalloped Potatoes/Vegetable Classics				
(Del Monte) microwave	4.5 oz	9	140	58%
Hash Browns/frozen-generic				
plain	½ cup	8.97	170	48%
(Kraft) Box Mixes-prepared				
Broccoli Au Gratin	½ cup	5	150	30%
Potatoes & Cheese	½ cup	4	130	28%
Mashed/w/whole milk	½ cup	.6	81	7%
w/whole milk & margarine	½ cup	4	94	38%
Instant Mix-Prepared				
(Hungry Jack)	½ cup	7	140	45%
(Micromagic) Frozen				
Crinkle Cut	3 oz	10.5	220	43%
French Fries	3 oz	13	290	40%
Microwave/(Ore Ida) frozen				
Cottage Fries	3 oz	4	130	38%
Crinkle Cuts, Microwave	3.5 oz	8	190	40%
French Fries-Golden Fries	3 oz	3	120	23%

Food and Description	Amount	Fat Grams	Total Calories	% Fat Calories
Hash Browns-Toaster	1.75 oz	5	100	54%
Tater Tots/Regular	3 oz	8	160	42%
Top Baked/Broccoli & Cheese	5⅞ oz	4	160	23%
(Pillsbury) box mixes/prepared				
Cheddar & Bacon	1 serv	5	130	35%
Potato Pancake	3 cakes	2	90	20%
Sour Cream & Chives	1 serv	7	150	42%
Potato Fillets/frozen				
(Gorton's)	2 fillets	20	310	58%
Potato Pancakes				
(French's) /Box Mix	3 cakes	2	90	20%
Potato Puffs/frozen	1 puff	.8	16	45%
Potato Sticks/Frozen (Gorton's)	4 sticks	16	260	55%
POTATO SNACKS				
(Keebler) Tato Skins-all flavors	1 oz	8	150	48%
Potato Sticks-Generic	1 cup	12	190	57%
PRETZELS				
(Eagle)/Plain	1 oz	2	110	16%
(Nabisco)/Mister Salty				
Butter Flavored	1 oz	1	110	8%
Pretzel Rings	1 oz	2	110	16%
Pretzel Sticks	1 oz	1	90	10%
Very Thin Pretzel Sticks	1 oz	1	110	8%
(Planter's) Pretzels	1 oz	1	110	8%
(Rold Gold)/Bavarian	1 oz	2	120	15%
Rods	1 oz	2	110	16%
Twists	1 oz	1	110	8%
(Snyder's) Hard Pretzels				
Old Fashioned	1 oz	0	110	0
(Ultra Slim Fast)	1 oz	<1	100	5
PRUNE				
Generic/canned in heavy syrup	1 cup	<1	240	2%
cooked/dried-no sugar	1 cup	<1	225	2%
(Sunsweet) dried/bite size	2 oz	0	120	0
pitted	2 oz	0	140	0
PRUNE JUICE				
(Del Monte) unsweetened	6 oz	0	120	0
(Mott's) country style	6 oz	0	129	0

Food and Description	Amount	Fat Grams	Total Calories	% Fat Calories
PUDDING & MOUSSE				
Canned/Banana	1/2 cup	4	150	24%
Chocolate	1/2 cup	4	190	19%
Fudge	1/2 cup	4	190	10%
Tapioca	1/2 cup	4	140	26%
(Del Monte) Pudding Cups				
Butterscotch	5 oz	5	180	25%
Chocolate Fudge	5 oz	6	190	28%
Tapioca	5 oz	4	180	20%
Mix/(Jell-O) Instant - Prepared w/Whole Milk				
Chocolate	½ cup	4	130	28%
Vanilla	½ cup	4	140	26%
(Jell-O) Instant-Sugar Free-Prepared w/2% Low-Fat Milk				
Chocolate Fudge	½ cup	3	100	27%
Vanilla	½ cup	2	90	20%
(Jell-O) Microwave Puddings-Prepared w/Whole Milk				
Chocolate	½ cup	5	170	27%
Vanilla	½ cup	4	160	23%
(Jell-O) Regular Puddings-Prepared w/Whole Milk				
Butterscotch	½ cup	4	170	21%
Chocolate	½ cup	5	180	25%
Vanilla	½ cup	4	140	26%
(Jell-O) Regular Sugar-Free Puddings-Prepared w/2% Milk				
Chocolate	½ cup	3	90	30%
Vanilla	½ cup	2	80	23%
(Jell-O) Mousse-Rich & Luscious-Prepared w/Whole Milk				
Chocolate	½ cup	6	150	36%
(Jell-O) Rice Pudding				
Americana w/Whole Milk	½ cup	4	170	21%
(My-T-Fine) Dry Mix to Make ½ Cup Serving				
Almond	.9 oz	1	100	9%
Chocolate	.9 oz	0	100	0
(Royal) Instant Pudding/Butterscotch				
Prepared w/Whole Milk	½ cup	5	180	25%
Chocolate				
Prepared w/Whole Milk	½ cup	4	190	19%
(Weight Watchers) Instant-Prepared w/Skim Milk				
Chocolate	1/2 cup	0	100	0

Food and Description	Amount	Fat Grams	Total Calories	% Fat Calories
Vanilla	1/2 cup	0	90	0
Snack				
(Hershey's) Chocolate Bar Flavor-in the dairy case				
Chocolate	4 oz	6	180	30%
(Hershey's) Chocolate Bar Flavor, Free (fat-free)				
Chocolate Fudge	4 oz	0	100	0
Kisses	4 oz	0	100	0
(Jell-O) in the Dairy Case				
Chocolate	4 oz	6	170	32%
Vanilla	4 oz	7	180	35%
(Swiss Miss) Light-Pudding Snacks				
Chocolate	4 oz	2	100	18%
Vanilla	4 oz	1	100	9%
(Swiss Miss) Original-Pudding Snacks				
Butterscotch	4 oz	6	180	30%
Chocolate Fudge	4 oz	6	220	16%
Tapioca	4 oz	5	160	28%
(Ultra Slim Fast)/Chocolate	4 oz	< 1	100	5%
Vanilla	4 oz	< 1	100	5%
(Yoplait) Pudding Snacks				
Milk Chocolate	4 oz	4	170	21%
Vanilla	4 oz	4	150	24%
Tapioca Canned	5 oz	5	160	28%
(Jell-O) Americana Prepared w/Whole Milk				
Chocolate	½ cup	5	170	27%
Vanilla	½ cup	4	160	23%
PUDDING POPS				
(Jell-O) Pudding Pops				
Chocolate	1	2	80	23%
Chocolate-Covered Vanilla	1	7	130	49%
Vanilla	1	2	70	26%
PUMPKIN SEEDS				
dried/hulled	1 oz	13	155	75%
whole-roasted	1 oz	5.5	127	39%

R

Food and Description	Amount	Fat Grams	Total Calories	% Fat Calories
RAISIN				
Golden/seedless	1 cup	.75	453	2%
(Del Monte)	3 oz	0	260	0
(Sun Maid)	1/2 cup	0	260	0
RASPBERRY				
Black/canned in water	1 cup	2	110	16%
fresh	1 cup	2	100	18%
Red/canned in heavy syrup	1 cup	< 1	234	2%
fresh	1 cup	.66	61	10%
frozen/Lite Syrup (Birds Eye)	5 oz	< 1	90	5%
sweetened	1 cup	< 1	256	2%
RAVIOLI				
Canned, Beef/(Chef Boyardee)	7 oz	5	180	25%
(Franco-American)	7.5 oz	4.7	223	19%
Raviolio's-canned	7.5 oz	8	250	29%
w/ Meat Sauce	7.5 oz	10.8	284	34%
RELISH				
(Heinz)/Hamburger relish	1 oz	0	30	0
Hot Dog relish	1 oz	0	35	0
Sweet relish	1 Tbs	0	12	0
(Vlasic)/ Hot Dog relish	1 oz	<1	40	11%
RICE				
Long Grain/cooked	1/2 cup	0	90	0
Long Grain & Wild Rices				
Brown & Wild/dry	1/2 cup	1	130	7%
prepared w/ butter	1/2 cup	4	150	24%
Chicken Stock Sauce/dry	1/2 cup	2	140	13%
prepared w/ butter	1/2 cup	5	160	28%
(Minute Rice)				
Boil in Bag/prepared	1/2 cup	0	90	0
Brown/instant/prepared	½ cup	1	120	8%
White/prepared	⅔ cup	< 1	120	4%

Food and Description	Amount	Fat Grams	Total Calories	% Fat Calories
(Success)/Brown				
Biol in Bag/prepared	1/2 cup	0	103	0
10 Minute/prepared	1/2 cup	0	103	0
Natural Long Grain				
pre-cooked/prepared	1/2 cup	<1	90	5%
(Uncle Ben's)				
Boil In Bag/as packaged	½ cup	< 1	90	5%
White/cooked/long grain				
cold	1 cup	< 1	158	3%
hot	1 cup	< 1	223	2%
RICE CAKES				
■ STANDARD SIZE RICE CAKES				
(Hain)/5-Grain	1	<1	40	11%
Palin/Regular	1	<1	40	11%
Popcorn/White Cheddar	1	1	45	20%
(Quaker)/Corn				
White Cheddar	1	0	40	0
Low Sodium, Plain & Wheat	1	0	35	0
(Westbrae Natural)/Sesame	1	< 1	30	15%
RICE DISHES				
(Birds Eye) International Rice Recipes				
frozen/Italian Style	3.3 oz	1	120	8%
Spanish Style	3.3 oz	0	110	0
(Country Inn) as packaged w/o butter				
Broccoli Rice Au Gratin	1/2 cup	3	130	21%
Chicken Stock Rice	1/2 cup	1	130	7%
(Country Inn) 10 Minute Recipes as packaged w/o butter				
Broccli Almondine	1/2 cup	2	130	14%
Cauliflower Au Gratin	1/2 cup	3	130	21%
Homestyle Chicken & Veg.	1/2 cup	3	140	19%
(Golden Grain) Rice-A-Roni				
Prepared/Beef Flavor	½ cup	4	140	26%
Chicken Flavor	½ cup	4	150	24%
Chicken & Broccoli	½ cup	3	150	18%
Long Grain & Wild				
Original	½ cup	3	130	21%
Rice Pilaf	½ cup	4	150	24%

Food and Description	Amount	Fat Grams	Total Calories	% Fat Calories
Yellow	1/2 cup	4	140	26%
(Golden Grain) Rice-A-Roni				
Savory Classics/prepared				
Broccoli Au Gratin	½ cup	9	180	45%
Chicken & Broccoli Dijon	1 serving	5	160	28%
Garden Pilaf	1/2 cup	4	140	26%
Oriental Stir Fry	½ cup	6	150	34%
Zesty Cheddar	1/2 cup	7	180	40%
(Green Giant)				
One Serving Vegetables/frozen				
Rice Medley	4.5 oz	4	130	28%
Rice Originals/frozen				
Rice Medley	1/2 cup	1	100	9%
Rice w/ Herb Butter Sauce	1/2 cup	5	150	30%
(Hain) 3-Grain Side Dishes				
Chicken Meatless Style	1/2 cup	4	130	28%
Rice Oriental	1/2 cup	5	130	35%
(Heinz)/Beef Falvored/dry	1 oz	0	100	0
Chicken Flavored/dry	1 oz	1	100	9%
Spanish/canned	7.25 oz	5	150	30%
Spanish Pilaf/dry	1 oz	0	100	0
(La Choy)				
Chinese Fried Rice/canned	¾ cup	1	190	5%
(Lipton) Golden Saute (as packaged)				
Beef Flavor Fried Rice	½ cup	2	125	14%
Chicken Flavor Fried Rice	1/2 cup	2	130	14%
Rice & Sauce/Beef	1/4 pkg	<1	120	4%
Broccoli & Cheddar	1/4 pkg	2	125	14%
Chicken	1/4 pkg	1	125	7%
Mushroom	1/4 pkg	<1	123	4%
(Minute Rice)				
Fried-prepared w/oil	½ cup	5	160	28%
Long Grain & Wild-prepared w/ butter	½ cup	4	150	24%
(Suzi Wan) Stir Fry Broccoli mix	1 serving	3	200	14%
w/added ingredients	7.5 oz	15	370	37%
Teriyaki mix	1 serving	1	180	5%
w/added ingredients	7.5 oz	12	360	30%

Food and Description	Amount	Fat Grams	Total Calories	% Fat Calories
ROLLS				
Brown & Serve/(Country Hearth) Krusty Rolls				
Italian	1	4	170	21%
(Pepperidge Farm) frozen				
Butter Crescent	1	6	110	49%
Club Enriched	1	1	100	9%
(Wonder)				
Crusty Italian Rolls du Jour	1	1	80	11%
Butterflake-refrigerated				
(Pillsbury)	1	5	140	32%
Dinner/(Pepperidge Farm)	1	2	60	30%
Country Style Classic	1	1	50	18%
(Wonder)	1	1	80	11%
Garlic Rolls-frozen/(Cole's)	1	5	100	45%
Kaiser/(Brownberry) Hearth	1	2	110	16%
Onion (Earth Grains)	1	2	190	10%
Pan (Wonder)	1	1	80	11%
Popover/mix	1	5	170	27%
Potato Roll	1	2	130	14%
Rye	1	0	87	0
Sandwich Rolls/(Pepperidge Farm)				
Frankfurter Enriched	1	3	140	19%
Sandwich Buns				
w/ sesame seeds	1	3	140	19%
Soft Hoagie	1	5	210	41%
(Weight Watchers)				
Hamburger and/or Hot Dog	1	< 1	80	6%
(Wonder)/Hamburger Buns	1	2	120	15%
Light	1	1	80	11%
Hoagie Rolls	1	7	400	16%
Hot Dog Rolls	1	1	80	11%
Sourdough	1	1	130	7%
Wheat Dinner Rolls (Home Pride)	1	1	70	13%
White-soft				
hamburger and/or hotdog	1	2	150	12%
hotdog (Wonder)	1	1	80	11%
White-soft dinner (Home Pride)	1	2	80	23%
Whole Wheat	1	1	93	10%

S

Food and Description	Amount	Fat Grams	Total Calories	% Fat Calories
SALAD DRESSING				
■ **MIXES & HOME RECIPE**				
(NOTE: Mixes were prepared as directed on package.)				
Bleu Cheese & Herbs				
(Good Seasons)	1 Tbs	8	70	100%
Blue Cheese/Chunky	1 Tbs	8	75	96%
(Hidden Valley)	1 Tbs	6	58	93%
Cheese Garlic (Good Seasons)				
Prepared	1 Tbs	8	70	100%
Creamy Italian-Fat Free (Good Seasons)				
w/regular mayonnaise	1 Tbs	1	16	56%
French, Thick 'n Creamy	1 Tbs	9	100	81%
(Hidden Valley) Prepared				
Creamy Herb	1 Tbs	6	58	93%
Ranch w/ Bacon/Regular	1 Tbs	3	35	77%
Honey Mustard-Fat Free				
(Good Seasons)/Prepared	1 Tbs	1	18	50%
Italian (Good Seasons)	1 Tbs	8	70	100%
Italian-Zesty				
(Good Seasons)/Lite	1 Tbs	3	25	100%
Regular	1 Tbs	8	70	100%
Ranch (Good Seasons)/Lite	1 Tbs	2	30	60%
Regular	1 Tbs	6	60	90%
■ **READY TO USE**				
Bacon, Creamy				
(Kraft) reduced calorie	1 Tbs	2	30	60%
(Bertolli) Original Olive Oil	1 Tbs	8	80	90%
Blue Cheese Chunky				
(Kraft)/Reduced calorie	1 Tbs	2	30	60%
(Wish Bone)/Lite	1 Tbs	4	40	90%
Buttermilk, Creamy (Kraft)				
Reduced Calorie	1 Tbs	3	30	90%

Food and Description	Amount	Fat Grams	Total Calories	% Fat Calories
Regular	1 Tbs	8	80	90%
Buttermilk Recipe (Seven Seas)				
Light	1 Tbs	1	50	18%
Regular	1 Tbs	8	80	90%
Caesar (Wish Bone)				
Catalina French (Kraft)				
Reduced calorie	1 Tbs	1	18	50%
Regular	1 Tbs	5	60	75%
Cucumber, Creamy/(Kraft)				
Reduced calorie	1 Tbs	2	25	72%
Regular	1 Tbs	8	70	100%
Dijon, Creamy (Estee)	1 Tbs	<1	8	56%
Dijon Vinaigrette-Classic (Wish Bone)				
Regular	1 Tbs	6	60	90%
French(Kraft) Miracle				
Reduced calorie	1 Tbs	1	20	45%
Regular	1 Tbs	6	60	90%
French, Red (Wish Bone)				
Original	1 Tbs	6	65	83%
Garlic, Creamy (Kraft)	1 Tbs	5	50	90%
(Wish Bone)	1 Tbs	8	74	97%
(Hain) Canola Oil Dressings				
Garden Tomato Vinaigrette	1 Tbs	6	60	90%
Creamy Caesar	1 Tbs	6	60	90%
Thousand Island	1 Tbs	5	50	90%
Traditional Italian	1 Tbs	8	80	90%
(Hidden Valley)				
Cole Slaw Dressing	1 Tbs	16	160	90%
Original Creamy	1 Tbs	6	80	90%
Italian, Creamy				
(Kraft)/Reduced calorie	1 Tbs	2	25	72%
(Wish Bone) Lite	1 Tbs	2	25	70%
Regular	1 Tbs	5	55	82%
Italian w/ Olive Oil				
(Seven Seas) Light	1 Tbs	3	30	90%
(Wishbone)	1 Tbs	3	33	83%
(Miracle Whip)/Cholesterol-free	1 Tbs	7	70	90%
Light	1 Tbs	4	45	80%

Food and Description	Amount	Fat Grams	Total Calories	% Fat Calories
Ranch/(Wish Bone)/Lite	1 Tbs	4	45	80%
Original	1 Tbs	8	80	90%
Russian/(Kraft)				
Reduced calorie	1 Tbs	1	30	30%
Regular	1 Tbs	5	60	75%
(Seven Seas) Buttermilk Recipe Ranch				
Regular	1 Tbs	8	80	90%
Viva-Herbs & Spices/Lite	1 Tbs	3	30	90%
Thousand Island/(Kraft) Regular	1 Tbs	5	60	75%
(Wish Bone)				
Lite	1 Tbs	< 1	20	23%
Regular	1 Tbs	6	60	90%
SALAD TOPPINGS				
(McCormick/Schilling)				
Bac'n Pieces/Bits	1 Tbs	< 1	25	18%
Cheese	1 Tbs	.7	31	20%
Garden Vegetable	1 Tbs	.7	34	19%
SALMON				
Pink/canned				
(Bumble Bee)	3.5 oz	8	160	45%
(Chicken Of The Sea) spring	3.5 oz	2	97	19%
Smoked	3 oz	8	150	48%
SARDINES				
Atlantic/canned in Olive Oil				
(Crown Prince) Brislingl	3.75 oz	42	460	82%
Pacific/canned in mustard sauce				
(Underwood)	3.75 oz	16	220	66%
SAUCE				
■ DEHYDRATED MIXES				
Curry/Generic (1 oz)				
Prepared w/ milk	1 cup	14.7	270	49%
Hollandaise				
(Durkee) Prepared	3/4 cup	14	173	73%
(French's) Prepared	1/4 pkg	1	30	30%
Honey Mustard (Mayacamas)				
Prepared	1 Tbs	3	32	84%
Sour Cream/Generic (1.2 oz)				
Prepared w/ milk	1 cup	30	509	53%

Food and Description	Amount	Fat Grams	Total Calories	% Fat Calories
Spaghetti				
(Durkee)/Mushroom/Prepared	2 2/3 cups	.8	208	4%
Regular/Prepared	2 1/2 cups	1	224	4%
(French's)/Mushroom/Prepared	1/2 cup	4	100	36%
Regular/Prepared	1/2 cup	4	90	40%
Thick/Prepared	7/8 cup	7	170	37%
Stroganoff (Durkee)/Prepared	4 cups	285	3280	78%
Sweet & Sour/Generic-Prepared	1 cup	0	294	0
Taco (Old El Paso)	1 pkg	1	100	9%
Teriyaki Sauce-Generic/Prepared	1 Tbs	0	8	0
■ READY-TO-USE & HOMEMADE				
Barbecue (Hunt's)/Original	1 Tbs	< 1	20	23%
Chicken Tonight (Ragu) Simmer Sauce				
Creamy Chicken Primavera	4 oz	6	90	60%
Oriental Chicken	4 oz	1	70	13%
Clam Sauce generic/red	2 oz	1.6	41	35%
white	2 oz	4.8	61	71%
Dijonaisse/(Golden Dipt)	1 oz	4	52	69%
Horseradish/(Heinz)	1 Tbs	7	75	84%
Manwich (Hunt's)/Sauce only	2.5 oz	1	35	26%
Marinara (tomato)	4 oz	4	86	42%
Pizza/canned				
(Chef Boyardee) w/cheese	2.5 oz	2	50	36%
(Contadina)/Quick & Easy	¼ cup	1	30	30%
Spaghetti Sauce-Canned				
(Chef Boyardee) Origl w/meat	3.75 oz	3	80	34%
(Healthy Choice) Flav. w/Meat	4 oz	< 1	50	9%
(Hunt's) Chunky Style	4 oz	< 1	50	9%
Homestyle	4 oz	2	60	30%
Traditional	4 oz	2	70	26%
(Progresso) Clam/Red	½ cup	3	70	39%
White	½ cup	8	110	65%
Marinara	½ cup	5	90	50%
Spaghetti Sauce-Fresh Chilled				
(Contadina) Alfredo	4 oz	34	350	87%
Marinara	5 oz	4	80	45%
Spaghetti Sauce-From Jars				
(Chef Boyardee)/Meatless	4 oz	1	60	15%

Food and Description	Amount	Fat Grams	Total Calories	% Fat Calories
(Classico)/Di Napoli	4 oz	4	70	51%
(Prego)/Extra Chunky				
Garden Combination	4 oz	2	80	23%
Marinara	4 oz	6	100	54%
Regular	4 oz	5	130	35%
Tomato & Basil	4 oz	2	100	18%
(Ragu)/Chunky Garden Style				
Italian Garden Combo	4 oz	2	80	23%
Fresh Italian/Garden Medley	4 oz	3	80	34%
Sweet'n Sour Sauce/(Contadina)	4 oz	3	150	18%
Tartar/(Kraft)-Original	1 Tbs	5	50	90%
Tomato-Canned (Del Monte)	1 cup	1	70	13%
(Hunt's)/Italian	4 oz	2	60	30%
White Cream Sauce/canned	4 oz	9	118	69%
SAUSAGE				
Beef Breakfast Strips/(Sizzlean)	2 strips	5	70	64%
Cooked-smoked	1 oz	7.6	89	77%
Pork Sausage/brown & serve	1 link	5	50	90%
Links/frozen (Schwan's)	1 oz	10	110	82%
SCALLOP				
Mixed/breaded & fried	2 large	3	67	40%
SEA BASS				
breaded & fried	3 oz	7	176	36%
SEAFOOOD ENTREE/DINNER				
(NOTE: Serving sizes for box dishes are for prepared portions.)				
(Booth) frozen/Individually Wrapped Fillets				
Cod	4 oz	1	90	10%
Clams/Frozen-breaded & fried				
(Mrs. Paul's)	2.5 oz	13	240	49%
Clams, Crunchy Strips-frozen				
(Gorton's)	3.5 oz	22	330	60%
Fillets				
Microwave/crunchy-frozen	1 fillet	22	330	60%
Fish Cakes/frozen	1 reg	10.7	162	59%
Fish Fillets in Buttery Herb Sauce				
frozen-microwave (Gorton's)	6.25 oz	8	190	38%
Fish'N Chips-frozen (Swanson)	6.5 oz	18	370	44%
Fish Sticks-frozen (4"x2"x½")	1 stick	3	76	36%

Food and Description	Amount	Fat Grams	Total Calories	% Fat Calories
(Gorton's) Frozen				
Crispy Batter Sticks	4 sticks	14	210	60%
Crunchy Fish Fillets	2 fillets	20	320	56%
Fishmarket Fresh/cod	5 oz	1	110	8%
flounder	5 oz	1	110	8%
(Healthy Choice) breaded				
Frozen/2 Fillets	3.5 oz	5	160	34%
8 Sticks	2.4 oz	4	120	30%
(Lean Cuisine) frozen entrees				
Filet of Fish Divan	10⅜ oz	5	210	21%
Tuna Lasagna	9.75 oz	7	240	26%
(Mrs. Paul's) frozen				
Au Natural/Cod Fillets	5 oz	2	110	16%
Seafood Salad	3½ oz	10	160	56%
Shrimp/frozen/(Booth Light Entree)				
Fettucine Alfredo	10 oz	8	260	28%
Sole/frozen/w/ Wine Sauce				
(Gorton's)	6.5 oz	7	180	35%
Sole, Fillet of, frozen/(Le Menu)	10 oz	14	360	35%
Tuna Helper (Betty Crocker) Prepared				
Cheesy Noodles'n Tuna	1 serving	8	240	30%
Creamy Noodles 'n Tuna	1 serving	14	300	42%
Romanoff	1 serving	8	290	25%
SEASONINGS				
(A Taste of Thai)/(Durkee) Beefstew Seasoning				
Prepared	8 cups	134	3032	40%
Sloppy Joe Seasoning				
Original/Prepared	2.5 cups	97	1453	60%
(Lipton) Microeasy Mix				
Barbeque Style Chicken	¼ pkg	.5	108	4%
Hearty Beef Stew	¼ pkg	.5	70	6%
(Manwich) Sloppy Joe Mix	⅙ pkg	< 1	20	23%
(Shake & Bake)/Oven Fry Seasoned Coating Mix				
Chicken/Extra Crispy	¼ pouch	2	190	15%
SHERBET	1 cup	4	270	13%
(Sealtest)/Orange	½ cup	1	130	7%
SHORTENING				
(Crisco) Regular & Butter	1 Tbs	12	113	100%

Food and Description	Amount	Fat Grams	Total Calories	% Fat Calories
SHRIMP/ breaded & fried	3 oz	10	206	44%
SNACK CAKES				
(Drake's)				
All Butter Pound Cake	1 pkg	12	270	40%
Chocolate Chip Cookies	1 pkg	12	280	39%
Devil Dogs	1 pkg	16	360	40%
Fudge Brownies	1 pkg	15	380	36%
Oatmeal Cookies	1 pkg	8	240	30%
Pies/Apple	1 pkg	20	420	43%
Ring Ding	1 pkg	20	360	50%
Yankee Doodle	1 pkg	12	300	36%
Yodel	1 pkg	18	300	54%
(Hostess)				
Brownie Bites/Plain	5 pieces	15	260	52%
Crumb Cake	1 cake	4	160	23%
Crumb Coffee Cakes/Original	1 cake	5	120	38%
Cupcakes/Chocolate	1 cake	6	180	30%
Ding Dongs	1 cake	9	170	48%
Snoball	1 cake	4	150	24%
Suzy Q's	1 cake	10	250	36%
(Little Debbie)/Baked Apple Pies	3 oz	9	310	23%
Coffee Cake	1 piece	3	110	25%
Nutty Bar	1 piece	10	160	56%
Oatmeal Creme Pies	1.35 oz	8	170	42%
(Sara Lee)/All Butter Pound	1 cake	11	200	50%
Chocolate Fudge	1 cake	10	190	47%
Classic Cheesecake	1 cake	14	200	63%
(Tastykake)/Brownie	1 piece	14	340	37%
Cupcakes/Chocolate Cream	1 piece	4	120	30%
Vanilla Sugar Wafer	1 piece	2	35	51%
SNACK MIX				
(Pepperidge Farm)/Classic	1 oz	8	140	51%
(Ralston) Chex Mix Brand				
Golden Cheddar	1 oz	5	130	35%
Traditional	1 oz	5	120	38%
(Sunshine)/Cheez-it Party Mix	1 oz	5	130	30%
SNACKS				
(Bugles)/Plain	1 oz	8	150	48%

Food and Description	Amount	Fat Grams	Total Calories	% Fat Calories
(Cheetos)/Cheddar Valley	1 oz	9	160	51%
Crunchy	1 oz	9	150	54%
(Combos) Cracker Cheddar	1 oz	8	150	48%
Pizza-Cheese	1 oz	5	130	35%
Pretzel	1 oz	6	130	42%
(Crunch'N Munch)/Caramel	1.25 oz	5	160	28%
(Eagle)/Cheese Crunch	1 oz	10	160	56%
(Pepperidge Farm) Snack Sticks				
Pretzel	8 pieces	3	120	23%
Three Cheese	8 pieces	5	130	35%
(Planter's)/Cheez Balls				
Nacho Cheez	1 oz	10	160	56%
Pork skins (Baken-ets)				
Original	1 oz	10	160	56%
Snack Mix (Snyder's)	1 oz	5	130	35%
(Wise)/Cheez Doodles/Crunchy	1 oz	10	160	56%

SOUP

(NOTE: Condensed soups were prepared as directed on packaging w/water, unless otherwise stated. When prepared with milk, whole milk was used. If you use low-fat or skim milk, refer to the Quick Reference-Milk on next page to adjust your fat and calorie data. Ready-To-Serve (RTS) soups were heated as directed w/no added liquid.)

QUICK REFERENCE: MILK	Amount	Fat Grams	Total Calories	% Fat Calories
Whole	½ cup	4	75	48%
2% lowfat	½ cup	2.5	61	37%
1% lowfat	½ cup	1	55	16%
Skim ½ cup	–	45	–	–

■ SOUP-CANNED

Beef/(Campbell's)	1 cup	2	80	23%
(Progresso) ready-to-serve	9.5 oz	5	160	28%
Beef Minestrone (Progresso)	9.5 oz	5	170	26%
Beef Noodle/(Campbell's)	1 cup	3	70	39%

Food and Description	Amount	Fat Grams	Total Calories	% Fat Calories
Beef Vegetable				
(Progresso) Ready-to-Serve	9.5 oz	3	150	18%
Broccoli, Cream of				
(Pepperidge Farm)	5.3 oz	6	100	54%
(Campbell's)				
Healthy Request				
Condensed-Prepared				
Chicken Noodle	8 oz	2	60	30%
Chicken w/Rice	8 oz	2	60	30%
Vegetable	8 oz	2	90	20%
Ready-to-Serve				
Hearty Chicken Noodle	8 oz	2	80	23%
Hearty Minestrone	8 oz	3	90	30%
Hearty Vegetable	8 oz	3	110	25%
Cauliflower (Campbell's)				
Creamy Natural	1 cup	9	130	62%
Celery, Cream of/Generic				
prepared w/milk	1 cup	9.68	165	53%
prepared w/water	1 cup	5.59	90	56%
Chicken Alphabet (Campbell's)	1 cup	2	70	26%
Chicken Broth	1 cup	1	39	23%
(Campbell's)/Original	1 cup	2	35	51%
(Health Valley) Natural				
No Salt	7.5 oz	1.6	35	41%
Chicken, Cream of/(Campbell's)	1 cup	7	110	57%
Prepared w/Milk	1 cup	14.97	191	71%
Ready-to-Serve	7.27 oz	5.5	85	58%
Chicken Noodle/(Campbell's)				
Ready-to-Serve	7.27 oz	2	60	30%
Chicken Rice/Ready-to-serve				
(Campbell's)	7.27 oz	2	52	35%
(Progresso)	9.5 oz	3	130	21%
Clam Chowder-Manhattan				
(Campbell's)	1 cup	2	70	26%
Ready-to-Serve/(Progresso)	9.5 oz	2	120	15%
Clam Chowder-New England				
(Campbell's)	1 cup	3	80	34%
(Stouffer's) frozen	8 oz	9	180	45%

Food and Description	Amount	Fat Grams	Total Calories	% Fat Calories
Fat-free/(Hain)				
Chicken Broth	7.5 oz	< 1	100	5%
Split Pea & Carrots	7.5 oz	< 1	80	6%
Tomato Vegetable	7.5 oz	< 1	50	9%
(Health Valley)				
Beef Broth-No salt	6.9 oz	< 1	10	45%
Chicken Broth	6.9 oz	< 1	20	23%
French Onion/(Campbell's)	1 cup	2	60	30%
(Pepperidge Farm)	5.3 oz	4.7	71	60%
Lentil/(Progresso) RTS	9.5 oz	4	140	26%
(Lipton) Kettle Ready-frozen				
Boston Clam Chowder	6 oz	7	130	48%
Chicken Noodle	6 oz	2.9	94	28%
Minestrone/(Campbell's)	1 cup	2	80	23%
Mushroom, Cream of				
prepared w/milk	1 cup	13.59	203	60%
prepared w/water	1 cup	8.97	129	63%
Onion	1 cup	1.7	57	27%
Pea, Green/prepared w/milk	1 cup	7	239	26%
Tomato/(Campbell's)	1 cup	2	90	20%
(Pritikin)	7⅜ oz	.5	50	9%
Vegetable/(Campbell's)	1 cup	2	80	23%
(Health Valley)/Chunky	7.5 oz	7	120	52%
Natural-No Salt	7.5 oz	1	110	8%
(Progresso) Ready-to-Serve	9.5 oz	2	90	20%
Vegetable, Garden (Campbell's)	1 cup	1.8	63	26%
Won Ton/(Campbell's)	1 cup	1	40	23%

■ SOUP(DEHYDRATED)/MIX

(NOTE: Prepared as directed with water, unless otherwise stated. Pkg or cube servings are unprepared.)

Food and Description	Amount	Fat Grams	Total Calories	% Fat Calories
(Campbell's)/Microwaveable Cup (as packaged)				
Chicken Flavored Noodle	1.35 oz	3	140	19%
Hearty Noodle w/Vegetables	1.7 oz	2	180	10%
Celery, Cream of	1 cup	1.6	63	23%
Chicken Broth, Bouillon,				
Consomme	1 Pkg.	.8	16	45%
w/water	1 cup	1	21	43%
Chicken Noodle/(Campbell's)	1 cup	2	100	18%

Food and Description	Amount	Fat Grams	Total Calories	% Fat Calories
Clam Chowder-Manhattan	1 cup	1.55	65	22%
Clam Chowder-New England	1 cup	3.67	95	35%
(Lipton)/Cup-A-Soup				
Chicken & Noodles	6 oz	7	70	13%
Chicken-Flavored Broth	6 oz	.6	20	27%
Creamy Broccoli & Cheese	6 oz	4	70	51%
Onion	6 oz	.5	27	17%
Tomato	6 oz	.9	103	8%
Soup Mix/Chicken Noodle	8 oz	2	80	23%
Country Vegetable	8 oz	.7	80	8%
Soup Mix/Instant				
Beef Flavor Oriental	8 oz	1	180	5%
Chicken Flavor Oriental	8 oz	2	180	10%
(Lunch Bucket)/Microwaveable				
Beef Noodle	8.25 oz	1	120	8%
Chicken Noodle	8.25 oz	3	110	25%
Country Vegetable	8.25 oz	1	90	10%
Minestrone/(Manischewitz)	8 oz	1	70	6%
Mushroom	8 oz	4.86	96	46%
Vegetable/(Campbell's)	1 cup	1	60	15%
Vegetable, Cream of	1 cup	5.69	105	49%
SOUR CREAM				
(Kemp)	1 cup	42	450	84%
Cultured	1 oz	5	60	75%
Lite/Sour Cream	1 oz	2	30	6%
w/Chives	1 oz	5	60	75%
(Land O'Lakes)				
Lite/Plain	1 Tbs	2	40	45%
w/Chives	1 Tbs	2	40	45%
Regular	1 Tbs	3	30	90%
(Weight Watchers) Light	2 Tbs	2	35	51%
SOUR CREAM SUBSTITUTES				
Sour Cream-flavored sprinkle products				
Molly McButter	½ tsp	< 1	4	100%
Sour Cream/substitute				
non-butterfat	1 oz	4	42	86%
(Land O'Lakes)				
Light Dairy Blend	1 Tbs	1	20	45%

Food and Description	Amount	Fat Grams	Total Calories	% Fat Calories
SOYBEAN				
Green/boiled	½ cup	5.8	127	41%
(La Loma) canned w/liquid	~ 4 oz	7	120	53%
roasted	½ cup	21.8	405	48%
SPAGHETTI DINNER				
Spaghetti w/meat sauce				
Box (Kraft)	1 cup	14	360	35%
Canned (Franco-American)	7.5 oz	8	211	34%
Spaghetti w/meatballs & meat sauce				
Canned	1 cup	10	260	35%
(Chef Boyardee)	7.5 oz	9	230	31%
(Franco-American)	7⅜ oz	8	220	33%
Spaghetti w/meatballs & tomato sauce				
canned	1 cup	10.8	258	38%
Spaghetti w/tomato sauce & cheese				
canned	1 cup	1.5	190	7%
SPAGHETTIO'S				
Canned (Franco-American)				
w/Meat balls	7⅜ oz	8	210	34%
SPICE BLENDS				
(Lawry's)/Pinch of Herbs	1 tsp	.5	9	50%
(McCormick/Schilling)				
Sesame All-Purpose	1 tsp	1	15	60%
SPINACH DISHES				
Creamed Spinach/frozen				
(Birds Eye)	½ cup	4	60	60%
(Green Giant)	½ cup	3	70	39%
SQUASH DISHES				
Zucchini, Breaded/frozen (Ore Ida)	2.7 oz	8	150	48%
STRAWBERRY				
Fresh	1 cup	.56	45	11%
Generic-frozen/Sweetened				
Sliced	1 cup	< 1	245	2%
Unsweetened/Thawed	3.5 oz	< 1	50	9%
STUFFING				
(Betty Crocker)-mix				
Chicken/prepared	¼ pkg	9	180	45%
Traditional Herb/prepared	¼ pkg	8	180	40%

Food and Description	Amount	Fat Grams	Total Calories	% Fat Calories
(Stove Top Stuffing) Microwave				
Regular/prepared w/butter	½ cup	7	160	39%
prepared w/o butter	½ cup	4	130	28%
(Stove Top Stuffing) Mix-prepared w/butter				
Americana San Francisco	½ cup	9	170	48%
Chicken Flavor	½ cup	9	180	45%
Long Grain & Wild Rice	½ cup	9	180	45%
prepared w/o butter				
Chicken Flavor	½ cup	1	110	8%
SUNFLOWER NUTS				
(Planters)/dry roasted	1 oz	14	160	79%
unsalted	1 oz	15	170	79%
SUNFLOWER SEED				
(Frito Lay's)	1 oz	16	170	85%
(Planters)	1 oz	14	160	79%
SWEET POTATO				
boiled-no skin-mashed	½ cup	.5	172	3%
canned-mashed	1 cup	.5	258	2%
fresh-baked-mashed	½ cup	< 1	103	4%
frozen-baked	½ cup	< 1	88	5%
SWEET POTATO DISHES				
(Birds Eye) Specialty Classics				
Candied Sweet Potatoes	5 oz	9	220	37%

T

Food and Description	Amount	Fat Grams	Total Calories	% Fat Calories
TOFU				
dried-frozen	~ ½ oz	5	82	55%
fried	~ ½ oz	2.6	35	67%
Okara	½ cup	1	47	19%
raw-firm	¼ block	7	118	53%

Food and Description	Amount	Fat Grams	Total Calories	% Fat Calories
TOFU FROZEN DESSERT PRODUCTS				
(Tofutti)/Chocolate Supreme	4 oz	13	230	51%
Vanilla, Chocolate, Strawberry	4 oz	< 1	90	5%
TOMATO MARINARA SAUCE				
red	1 cup	8	171	42%
TOMATO PASTE				
canned/plain	½ cup	1	110	8%
canned Italian style	2 oz	1	65	14%
TORTILLA CHIPS				
(Doritos)/Cool Ranch	1 oz	7	140	45%
Lights/all flavors	1 oz	4	110	33%
Nacho Cheese	1 oz	7	140	45%
Traditional	1 oz	6	140	39%
(Eagle)/Cantina Tortilla Nacho	1 oz	8	150	48%
(Fritos)/Bar-B-Q	1 oz	9	150	54%
Original	1 oz	10	150	60%
(Health Valley)/Cheese	1 oz	10	160	56%
No Salt	1 oz	11	160	62%
(Pringles)/Mild Nacho Cheese	1 oz	7	140	45%
(Tostitos)/Traditional	1 oz	8	140	51%
White Corn Rejstaurant	1 oz	6	130	42%
(Wise)				
Bravos-Nacho Cheese Flavor	1 oz	8	150	48%
Corn Chips/Corn Crunchies	1 oz	10	160	56%
TROUT				
Rainbow/broiled w/ butter	3 oz	9	175	46%
cooked-dry heat	3 oz	3.66	129	26%
smoked	3 oz	3	153	18%
TUNA				
Light Chunk/canned in oil				
(Bumble Bee)	2 oz	12	160	68%
(Star Kist)	2 oz	13	150	78%
Light Chunk/canned in water				
(Chicken of the Sea)	2 oz	1	60	5%
(Star Kist)	2 oz	.5	60	8%
White-chunk/canned in water				
(Bumble Bee)	2 oz	2	70	26%

Food and Description	Amount	Fat Grams	Total Calories	% Fat Calories
White-solid/canned in oil				
(Star Kist) Prime Catch-Light	2 oz	13	150	78%
canned in water (Bumble Bee)	2 oz	2	70	26%
TUNA HELPER				
(Betty Crocker) prepared				
Creamy Noodles	⅕ pkg	14	300	42%
Fettuccine Alfredo	⅕ pkg	13	300	41%
TURKEY				
(NOTE: All turkey meat is roasted, unless otherwise stated.)				
all classes/meat, skin, giblets, and neck-roasted-				
1 whole turkey	~ 9 lb	379.97	8245	42%
dark meat w/skin	~ 2 lb	93	1789	47%
dark meat w/o skin	~ 5 oz	10	262	34%
light meat w/skin	2¼ lb	87	206	38%
light meat w/o skin	~ 5 oz	4.5	219	19%
meat only (dark & light)	~ 5 oz	6.95	238	26%
(Butterball)/boneless-light & dark-meat				
only-cooked	3.5 oz	7	140	45%
dark meat only-cooked	3.5 oz	7	175	36%
(Butterball) cooked parts w/o skin				
Breast Slices	3.5 oz	3.5	140	23%
Drumsticks	3.5 oz	7	175	36%
Thighs	3.5 oz	14	245	51%
Wings	3.5 oz	10.5	210	45%
(Louis Rich)/Fresh Turkey Cuts				
Turkey Breast-cooked	1 oz	2	45	40%
Turkey Breast Roast-cooked	1 oz	1	40	23%
Turkey Wings	1 oz	3	55	49%
Turkey Breast (Armour)				
Turkey Selects-boneless				
Breast Roast	3 oz	5	120	38%
Breast slices	3 oz	1	90	10%
Turkey/ground-packaged	2 oz	7	122	52%
(Armour) Golden Star-raw	1 oz	4	50	72%
(Armour) Turkey Selects	3 oz	6	120	45%
TURKEY ENTREE/DINNER				
Turkey & Gravy/frozen	5 oz	3.7	95	35%
Turkey Dijon/frozen (Lean Cuisine)	9.5 oz	5	230	20%

Food and Description	Amount	Fat Grams	Total Calories	% Fat Calories
Turkey (Louis Rich)-breaded-frozen				
Turkey Nuggets-prepared	~ 1 oz	4	65	55%
Turkey Pot Pies./frozen				
(Stouffer's)	10 oz	33	530	56%
(Swanson)/Hungry Man	16 oz	36	650	50%
TURKEY PRODUCTS				
Turkey Bacon (Armour)-Turkey Selects	1 strip	2	35	51%
Turkey Frankfurter-Generic	2.5 oz	8	102	71%
Turkey Pastrami	2 oz	3.5	80	39%
Turkey Roll/light	1 oz	2	42	43%

V

Food and Description	Amount	Fat Grams	Total Calories	% Fat Calories
VEAL CUTS				
Breast/lean & fat-braised	3 oz	18	258	63%
Chop/Lean & fat-fried				
w/ bone-raw	6.5 oz	18.6	282	59%
Lean only w/bone-raw	6.5 oz	6.6	177	34%
Chuck/lean & fat-cooked	3 oz	10.9	200	49%
Cutlet, Steak				
Lean & fat/Boneless-broiled				
braised	3 oz	9.4	182	47%
Lean only/Boneless-broiled				
braised	3 oz	3.5	140	23%
Ground or patty broiled				
(4 oz raw)	2.4 oz	8.9	156	51%
Rib Roast/lean & fat				
Roasted	3 oz	14	230	55%

VEAL DISHES
(NOTE: The data listed in this table may vary slightly, depending on the fat content of the veal cuts used in preparation.)

Food and Description	Amount	Fat Grams	Total Calories	% Fat Calories
Veal Parmigiana/Frozen				
(Banquet)/Breaded	5 oz	11	230	43%
w/Sauce & Cheese	~ 6.5 oz	18	282	57%
(Swanson's)	~ 12 oz	22	450	44%
Veal Patty Parmigiana				
Frozen (Weight Watchers)	8.44 oz	10	220	41%
VEAL STEAKS				
Frozen (Hormel)/Breaded	4 oz	13	240	49%
Unbreaded	4 oz	4	130	28%
VEGETABLE DISHES				
Broccoli, carrots, & pasta w/lightly seasoned sauce/frozen				
(Birds Eye)	⅔ cup	4	87	41%
Broccoli, Cauliflower, Carrots w/cheese sauce				
frozen/(Birds Eye)	5 oz	5	100	45%
Corn, green beans, & pasta curls w/light cream sauce				
frozen (Birds Eye)	½ cup	4.9	108	41%
Garden Salad/canned (Joan of Arc)	½ cup	0	70	0
Micro Quick/frozen (Freshlike)				
Broccoli, Pasta, Carrots in Cheese Sauce	4.5 oz	3	100	27%
Peas, Cauliflower, Red Peppers in Butter Sauce	5 oz	2	90	20%
Mixed vegetables in butter sauce				
frozen (Green Giant)	½ cup	2	60	30%
Vegetable Lasagna				
(Impromtu Lite) box mix-micro.	10.6 oz	11	290	34%
Vegetable Medley				
breaded/frozen (Ore Ida)	3 oz	9	160	51%
Vegetables in Creamy Cheese Sauce				
frozen (Birds Eye)Custom Cuisine	3.5 oz	5	210	21%
Vegetarian Medley/frozen (Kibun)	10 oz	2	240	8%
VEGETABLES, MIXED				
Succotash (lima beans & corn)				
(Libby)	½ cup	1	80	11%
w/Cream-Style Corn	½ cup	.7	102	6%
w/Whole Kernel Corn	½ cup	.6	81	7%

Food and Description	Amount	Fat Grams	Total Calories	% Fat Calories
Frozen (Birds Eye)				
Broccoli, carrots, & pasta twists	~ ½ cup	4	9	40%
Chow Mein Style - Int'l Recipe	~ ½ cup	4	90	40%
Corn, green beans, & pasta	~ ½ cup	5	110	41%
Pasta Primavera - Int'l Recipe	~ ½ cup	5	120	38%
(Green Giant) Microwaveable/Pantry Express				
Corn, Green Beans, Carrots, & Pasta	½ cup	2	80	23%
Mixed Vegetables	½ cup	1	35	26%
Cauliflower in Cheese-Flavored Sauce	5.5 oz	2	80	23%
Valley Combinations (Pillsbury/Green Giant)-Dual Pouch				
American Style w/sauce	½ cup	2	70	26%
Broccoli Cauliflower Medley w/sauce	½ cup	2	60	30%
Broccoli Fanfare w/sauce	½ cup	2	80	23%
VEGETARIAN FOOD				
(Amy's) Frozen/Country Dinner	11.35 oz	20	482	37%
Lasagna (Organic Vegetable)	10 oz	7	310	20%
Macaroni & Cheese	1 serving	10.8	226	43%
(La Loma) Canned & Dry Packed - Meatless				
Big Franks	1.8 oz	6	110	49%
Dinner Cuts	3.5 oz	1	110	49%
Redi-Burger	2.4 oz	6	130	42%
Vege-burger mix	½ cup	2	110	16%
Frozen Products - Meatless				
Chik Nuggets	5 pieces	20	270	67%
Fried Chicken	2 oz	14	180	70%
Sizzle Burger	2.5 oz	12	220	49%
(Worthington)				
Canned & Dry Packed - Meatless				
Chili	⅔ cup	10	190	47%
Country Stew	9.5 oz	10	220	47%
Frozen Products - Meatless				
Beef Pie-Vegetarian	8 oz	16	360	40%
Chicken/Diced	½ cup	13	190	62%
Chicken Pie-Vegetarian	8 oz	20	380	47%
Dinner Roast	2 oz	8	120	60%

Food and Description	Amount	Fat Grams	Total Calories	% Fat Calories
Egg Rolls-Vegetarian	1	6	160	34%
Natural Touch Dinner Entree	1 pattie	13	210	56%

W

Food and Description	Amount	Fat Grams	Total Calories	% Fat Calories
WAFFLE				
Box-Mix-/(Aunt Jemima)				
Buttermilk	⅓ cup	1	75	12%
Original	¼ cup	1	108	8%
Whole wheat	⅓ cup	1	142	6%
Frozen/(Aunt Jemima)				
Buttermilk	2.5 oz	5.8	179	29%
Lite	1 waffle	1	70	13%
Original	2.5 oz	5.6	173	29%
(Downyflake)/Hot-N-Buttery	2	6	180	30%
Multi-grain	2	14	250	50%
Plain/regular	2	3	120	23%
(Eggo)/Blueberry	1	5	130	35%
Buttermilk	1	5	120	38%
(Eggo/Nutri-Grain)/Plain	1	5	120	38%
Shake 'N Pour Mix (Bisquick)				
Original	2	6	280	19%
WALNUT				
Black/(Planters)	1 oz	17	180	85%
WATERMELON				
Fresh/10" diameter	1/16 wedge	2	152	12%
WHEAT GERM				
(Kretschmer)/Plain	¼ cup	3	100	27%
WHIPPED TOPPING				
frozen	1 Tbs	1	15	60%
frozen-non dairy	1 Tbs	.8	11	66%

Food and Description	Amount	Fat Grams	Total Calories	% Fat Calories
pressurized-cream	1 Tbs	1	8	100%
non dairy	1 Tbs	1	10	81%
WHITEFISH				
Mixed/(Mother's) jellied	1 fishball	1	46	20%
jellied in broth	1 fishball	1	70	13%
Smoked	3 oz	.79	92	8%
WHITEFISH & PIKE				
jar (Manischewitz)	3.5 oz	3.57	99	33%
jellied (Rokeach)	1 fishball	1	60	15%
WHITING				
breaded & fried	3 oz	9.7	171	51%
cooked-dry heat	3 oz	1	98	9%

Y

Food and Description	Amount	Fat Grams	Total Calories	% Fat Calories
YEAST				
Active dry/Baker's	1 oz	.5	80	6%
YOGURT, DAIRY				
(Breyers)/Black Cherry	8 oz	5	270	17%
Mixed Berry-low fat	8 oz	2	250	7%
Plain	8 oz	8	190	38%
Strawberry	8 oz	5	270	17%
Vanilla Bean	8 oz	7	230	27%
(Columbo) Lite/Coffee	8 oz	< 1	190	2%
Peach	8 oz	< 1	190	2%
Vanilla	8 oz	< 1	110	4%
(Del Monte) Yogurt Cup 1½% milkfat				
Rad Raspberry	4¾ oz	2	140	13%
Totally Strawberry	4¾ oz	2	140	13%
(Kemps) Vanilla & Fruit,	6 oz	2	160	11%
(La Yogurt) All fruit flavors	6 oz	4	190	19%

Food and Description	Amount	Fat Grams	Total Calories	% Fat Calories
Plain	6 oz	6	140	39%
(Light N'Lively) 99% fat free				
Blueberry	5 oz	1	150	6%
Strawberry Fruit Cup	5 oz	2	150	12%
Original/Blueberry	8 oz	2	240	8%
Strawberry	8 oz	2	240	8%
Lowfat/Coffee, Vanilla-lowfat	4 oz	1	97	9%
Fruit-lowfat	4 oz	1	115	8%
Plain-lowfat	4 oz	1.8	72	23%
(Weight Watchers)/all flavors	8 oz	1	150	6%
(Whitney's) Original/Plain	6 oz	7	150	42%
Strawberry Banana	6 oz	5	200	23%
Vanilla	6 oz	6	200	27%
(Yoplait) Custard style/Banana	6 oz	4	190	19%
Light/all flavors	6 oz	.5	90	5%
Low Fat/Strawberry-Banana	6 oz	4	240	15%
Original/Mixed berry	6 oz	4	190	19%
Vanilla	6 oz	3	180	15%
YOGURT BARS				
(Kemps) Yogurt Dipped On A Stick				
Vanilla	1 bar	7	120	53%
YOGURT DESSERT (Sara Lee)				
Frozen strawberry-light	1 slice	< 1	120	4%
YOGURT DRINKS				
(Dannon) All flavors	8 oz	4	190	19%
(Weight Watchers)/Frozen				
Chocolate	7.5 oz	1	220	4%
YOGURT, FROZEN				
(Dannon) On A Stick-All flavors	1.75 oz	1	50	18%
(Danny) Yogurt Bars				
Chocolate-chocolate coated	1 bar	8	130	55%
Vanilla	1 bar	1	60	15%
(Dreyer's) Inspirations				
Low-fat/Chocolate	3 oz	1	80	11%
Vanilla	3 oz	1	80	11%
(Haagen-Dazs)/Chocolate	4 oz	4	170	21%
Vanilla almond crunch	4 oz	6	190	28%
(Sealtest)/Black cherry	1/4 pint	2	120	15%

Food and Description	Amount	Fat Grams	Total Calories	% Fat Calories
Strawberry	1/4 pint	2	110	16%
(Yoplait)/Chocolate	4 oz	3	130	21%
Vanilla	4 oz	3	120	23%

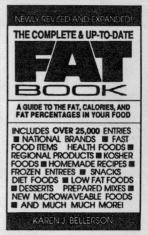